The Secret to Alzheimer's Dementia Care

Learn to Manage Challenging and Aggressive Behaviors, Reduce Stress and Burnout, and Gain Essential Knowledge to Be a Confident, Compassionate Caregiver

Renée Remy

DOVETAIL EDUCATION

For permission requests and speaking inquiries, and bulk order purchase options, email: support@dovetailedu.com.

1st edition 2024
Published by Dovetail Education

ISBN: 978-1-965952-02-3 | E-book

ISBN: 978-1-965952-00-9 | Paperback

ISBN: 978-1-965952-01-6 | Hardcover

This book is dedicated to

the patients and families I have had the honor to care for

the Hospice and Palliative Care teams I have been blessed to worked with

my editor, without whom, this book would never have been completed

the friends who are always there for me when I pick up the phone

and my family who are always supportive

I am grateful for all of you!

Table of Contents

Section Three
Compassionate Care

Section Four
Navigating the Caregiver's
Emotional Journey

Section Five
Legal and Financial Planning

Section Six
Innovations in Alzheimer's Care

Section Seven
Honoring Your Loved One's Legacy

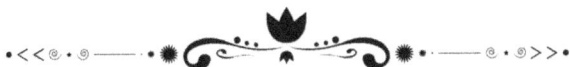

Just for you!

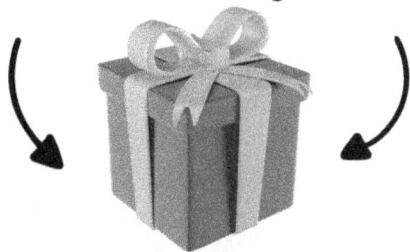

A Free Gift For Our Readers

Empower Yourself to Confidently Communicate with your Alzheimer's Care professionals!
Over 140 essential terms plus more!

Scan the QR Code or visit the link below.

https://bit.ly/empowered-caregiver

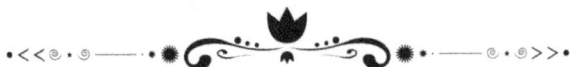

Introduction

During one of those quiet afternoons that blended into our routine, I sat beside my mother, her hands folded loosely in her lap, eyes gazing out to the garden. I remember reading aloud from her favorite novel, her face suddenly brightening with recognition at a familiar passage. This moment, fleeting and precious, captured the essence of our journey through Alzheimer's—a path marked by challenges but also filled with moments of profound connection. It's in these moments that the true nature of caregiving reveals itself—not just as a duty but as an intimate dance of love and patience.
—Terry

My role as a Hospice and Palliative Care Chaplain has given me the privilege of supporting numerous individuals through the challenges and joys of caring for loved ones with dementia, as well as working with the patients directly. These experiences provided me with extensive training in helping families manage the journey of dementia and the unique difficulties of Alzheimer's disease. It was through caring for my mother, however, that I encountered the deep, personal impact of Alzheimer's. These dual experiences have equipped me not only with professional insights, but also a profound understanding of the emotional and practical complexities faced by caregivers.

This book comes from a place of compassion, empathy, and a passionate desire to help those who are struggling with the frustration, overwhelm, burnout, guilt, and anxiety that comes with caring for a loved one diagnosed with Alzheimer's. It is inspired by the many caregivers who desire to provide loving and compassionate care, and the information I wish I had known before I started my own caregiving journey.

It's designed to guide you, the caregiver, through the multifaceted challenges of Alzheimer's care. From preparing the foundation that will ease the transitions through the stages of this disease, to navigating the behavioral changes that seem sudden and mystifying, to handling legalities and finding emotional support, I hope this manual equips you with the knowledge, practical advice, and resources that you need. More than that, I hope it strengthens your emotional resilience, and sustains your well-being while you provide the best compassionate care that you can.

Caring for someone with Alzheimer's is an emotional journey. One that might find you grappling with a confusing mix of feelings—ranging from isolation, frustration, sorrow, and even joy and satisfaction. This book acknowledges the complexity of these competing emotions and offers itself as a source of comfort and community.

I share real life scenarios from my experiences and the experiences of others who have cared for loved ones with Alzheimer's, and the solutions that worked for them. My hope is to bridge the gap between clinical advice and the realities of daily care, ensuring you have access to relatable and effective strategies.

There's no one solution that is perfect for every caregiver. Use the practical advice, foundational guidance, and stories to help you tailor the strategies to your own situation. As you apply and adapt these strategies, you'll soon find that the secret to navigating this journey is three-fold. I'll leave clues to this secret as we go along, and by the end, we'll see if you've discovered them on your own.

Structured to reflect the progressive stages of Alzheimer's, this book begins with a comprehensive description of the disease, followed by stage-specific care strategies that respect the dignity of your loved one while addressing some of the more difficult mood and behavioral changes. You'll learn all about compassionate care and how different techniques and tools can help you support your loved one effectively.

The section on caregiving is designed to cover both how to build resilience while on the emotional roller coaster of caregiving, and tips to tools to relieve some of the burden of caregiving.

As you turn these pages, you're encouraged not just to read, but to actively adapt and apply the insights and strategies to improve your caregiving journey. My hope is that you will see improvements in the quality of life for both you and your loved one long before you finish this book. When your loved one seems to be progressing to new symptoms or stages, you should be able to quickly refer to the section that addresses these changes to refresh your memory and support your new experiences.

You are not alone on this path. Together, we can navigate the complexities of Alzheimer's care, supporting our loved ones better due to the knowledge, compassion, and resilience we've acquired. Let's embark on this journey together, with hearts open and spirits ready to learn and grow.

Section One
Overview of Alzheimer's Disease

When my mother first began to forget little things—names of family members, where she left her glasses—we all laughed with her and brushed it off as signs of normal aging. She would sometimes joke about losing her memory, but we all thought it was just a figure of speech. However, it wasn't long before these memory slips grew into more concerning lapses, like forgetting to pay bills, or not recognizing certain items in the house that had belonged to her for years. It was during this troubling time that I realized how crucial it was to understand the nuances of her condition.

Whether you're noticing the initial, inconspicuous changes of your loved one, or are managing deeper stages of their condition, grasping the fundamentals of dementia and Alzheimer's disease is the first step in providing compassionate and effective care.

Understanding Dementia and Alzheimer's Disease

Dementia is not a specific disease but rather a broad term. It refers to a range of symptoms associated with memory decline and impaired cognitive function, significantly affecting a person's ability to perform everyday activities. Alzheimer's disease is one of the most common forms of dementia in the world, estimated to represent about 60-80% of all dementia cases. Picture dementia as a tree, where each branch represents different diseases such as Alzheimer's, vascular dementia, and Lewy body dementia.

Globally, the impact of dementia is staggering, with around 50 million people living with the condition and nearly 10 million new cases diagnosed every year. As the leading type of dementia, Alzheimer's disease not only strains healthcare systems but also deeply affects families emotionally and financially. It's a condition that progressively impairs the individual, demanding higher levels of care and supervision over time.

Causes of Alzheimer's

The underlying causes of Alzheimer's include a combination of lifestyle, environmental, and genetic factors that gradually affect the brain. Alzheimer's is characterized by the build-up of amyloid proteins clumping together to form "amyloid plaques" and tau proteins binding together inside nerve cells to create "tau tangles" in the brain. These amyloid plaques and tau tangles disrupt cell function, causing cells to die off. This results in brain shrinkage and the loss of connections between nerve cells, hindering cognitive and functional abilities.

Risk Factors

Risk factors for developing Alzheimer's range from modifiable factors like hypertension, obesity, and smoking, to non-modifiable factors such as age and genetics. While genetic predisposition cannot be altered, strategies that focus on improving cardiovascular health, maintaining a healthy diet, engaging in regular physical activity, and participating in activities that stimulate the brain can potentially reduce the risk of cognitive decline.

Diagnosing Alzheimer's Disease

Diagnosing Alzheimer's disease is a detailed process that involves evaluating an individual's medical history, conducting physical and neurological exams, and administering mental status tests. Brain imaging technologies such as magnetic resonance imaging (MRI) or computed tomography (CT) scans are often used to rule out other conditions that could mimic dementia symptoms, like normal pressure hydrocephalus or brain tumors.

Receiving an accurate and timely diagnosis of Alzheimer's is essential, as it opens the door to early interventions that can slow the progression of symptoms, enabling more effective planning for the future, and providing families with clarity and direction in managing the condition. If there's any uncertainty about the diagnosis, seeking a second opinion from a dementia specialist can be a valuable step to ensure that the assessment is thorough and accurate. This proactive approach can significantly impact how the disease is managed, helping to align the care provided with the individual's specific needs and stages of their condition.

Recognizing and grasping the nuances of dementia and Alzheimer's not only improves your understanding of these conditions, but also prepares you to handle the challenges of caregiving with an informed and confident stance. This foundational knowledge will be your guide in caregiving, whether you're having discussions with doctors, planning daily activities for your loved one, or explaining changes to family and friends.

The Seven Stages of Alzheimer's Disease

Alzheimer's disease progresses through seven stages, often grouped into three distinct categories: Early (Mild), Middle (Moderate), and Late (Severe). Each stage reflects the increasing severity of the disease and presents unique challenges for caregivers. Understanding these stages helps caregivers set realistic expectations and prepare for the journey ahead.

Early or Mild Stages (Stages 1-3)

Stages 1-3 cover the early stages of Alzheimer's dementia. In these stages, symptoms may be subtle and easily mistaken for normal age-related forgetfulness.

Stage 1: Barely Noticeable Decline

- **Duration**: Several years
- **Symptoms**: Often undetectable

  o No noticeable memory problems

    ○ Symptoms are discounted as normal

Stage 2: Very Mild Decline

- **Duration**: 2-4 years.
- **Symptoms**: These lapses are usually not evident to others, but may be to family members and your loved one

    ○ Slight memory lapses
    ○ Forgetting familiar words
    ○ Forgetting where everyday objects are located

Stage 3: Mild Decline

- **Duration**: 2-7 years.
- **Symptoms**: Noticeable difficulties with memory and thinking

    ○ Forgetting names or recent events
    ○ Challenges in social or work settings
    ○ Struggling to find the right words during conversations
    ○ Forgetting to pay bills
    ○ Forgetting to read mail

Caregiver Strategies for the Early Stages

During the early stages of Alzheimer's, caregivers might notice subtle changes in a person's behavior and memory. While these changes may not seem significantly impactful to daily life, they still require patience and understanding. Caregivers may want to focus on the following:

- **Encouraging Independence:** Assist your loved one only when necessary, encouraging them to maintain their usual routines and daily activities.
- **Using Organizational and Memory Aids:** Helping your loved one implement tools like calendars, reminders, and notes can help maintain organization and facilitate memory based activities.
- **Fostering Engagement:** Help your loved one stay engaged with socially and mentally stimulating activities.
- **Establishing Routines**: Start to establish routines for bill paying, meal prep, and other daily activities that partner with someone who may manage those routines in the future. This will create a sense of safety and familiarity that will stay with your loved one as the disease progresses.
- **Engaging in End of Life Conversations**: Speak to your loved one about who will make medical and financial decisions when they cannot, and their end of life preferences, like Do Not Resuscitate orders and burial/cremation preferences. Complete legal documentation and pre-planning documents as needed.

Middle or Moderate Stages (Stages 4-5)

Stages 4 and 5 mark the middle stages of Alzheimer's, where symptoms become more pronounced and challenging for caregivers. While the average duration of each stage is listed below, I've heard that the constant movement that may accompany this stage can last anywhere from 2-10 years.

Stage 4: Moderate Decline

- **Duration**: 2-3 years.
- **Symptoms**: Clear-cut symptoms such as:

○ Forgetting recent events or personal history
○ Wandering
○ Constant movement
○ Sundowning
○ Anxiety and Worrying
○ Agitation and Aggressiveness
○ Hallucinations, Delusions, and/or Paranoia that increase fear and agitation
○ Difficulty managing finances and complex tasks
○ Withdrawal from social situations
○ Easily Distracted
○ Hoarding Food and other objects
○ Difficulty focusing on reading and listening to music
○ Increasing difficulty with reading comprehension
○ Substituting words with something that does not make sense
○ Repetition of conversations becomes more frequent
○ Noticeably losing or gaining weight
○ Sleep cycle may be disrupted with increased hours of being awake, or they may sleep during the day and be awake at night

Stage 5: Moderately Severe Decline

- **Duration**: 1.5-2.5 years.
- **Symptoms**: Significant memory gaps emerge, and assistance with daily activities becomes necessary.

○ Confusion about time or place
○ Trouble remembering personal details like their address or phone number
○ Difficulty choosing appropriate clothing for the season or occasion

○ Increasing confusion in understanding and using language
○ Difficulty with physical activities like walking and fine motor skills like using silverware
○ Repetition of conversations happens more consistently

Caregiver Strategies for Middle Stages

In the middle stages, caregiving becomes increasingly more demanding as your loved one's cognitive abilities decline. This is the stage when caregivers can become frustrated and burned out quickly because there are so many new symptoms and routines that need to be changed or established. In addition, your loved one's increase in anxiety and need for safety, raises your anxiety. Caregivers can ease their burdens by doing the following:

- **Providing Structure:** Continue to implement daily routines that can be easily adjusted as the disease progresses. This helps reduce confusion and provide a sense of stability and normalcy.
- **Ensuring Safety:** Monitor and modify daily tasks such as cooking and cleaning to maintain a safe environment. Make sure your loved one cannot wander outside without you being alerted.
- **Ensuring Finances are Managed:** Transition the management of finances to a trusted person who can handle bills in a timely manner. File Power of Attorney documents with financial institutions as appropriate.
- **Communicating Effectively:** Use clear, simple communication to minimize frustration.
- **Showing Empathy and Compassion:** Use non-verbal communication to reduce agitation. Acknowledge feelings and distract (instead of arguing or correcting).

- **Finding Support:** Introduce new private caregivers or family caregivers for a few hours per week.
- **Improving Caregiver Self Care:** Have a daily routine for self-care, which includes allowing for adequate sleep, exercise, nutrition, and spiritual needs. Search for community resources or support groups to help relieve stress associated with caregiving. Establishing supportive relationships that you regularly nurture will make it easier to maintain those relationships, and your resilience, as caregiving becomes more demanding.

Late or Severe Stages (Stages 6-7)

Stages 6 and 7 encompass the severe stages of Alzheimer's dementia, where individuals require extensive care and support.

Stage 6: Severe Decline

- **Duration**: 1-2.5 years.
- **Symptoms**: As memory continues to worsen, significant changes in personality and physical capabilities may become more evident. Caregivers might notice the following symptoms in their loved ones:

  - Forgetting the names of close family members
  - Wandering and becoming lost
  - Needing assistance with basic personal care like dressing and toileting
  - Increased behavioral changes, such as suspicion or repetitive behaviors
  - Decreasing motor skills for activities like walking and feeding oneself
  - "Pocketing" food. This is where they chew the food

and leave it in the pockets of their cheeks, or they may simply leave the food in the mouth without attempting to swallow it

Stage 7: Very Severe Decline

- **Duration**: 1.5-2.5 years.
- **Symptoms:** In the final stage, people with Alzheimer's may lose their ability to effectively communicate or respond to their surroundings. Caregivers may observe the following:

  - Loss of ability to speak and comprehend language
  - Inability to control physical movements, such as walking, standing, or sitting
  - Needs assistance with all daily activities
  - Difficulty swallowing
  - Increased vulnerability to infections
  - Needs assistance with all personal care routines
  - May no longer show emotions like smiling
  - Increased hours of sleep

Caregiver Strategies for Late Stages

In the late stages of Alzheimer's dementia, caregivers will be met with more intensive demands as the person they're caring for will need help with every aspect of daily life. Caregivers will want to do the following:

- **Ensure Safety and Comfort:** Adapt the home environment as needed to promote safety and familiarity, making changes as the individual's needs evolve.

- **Communicate Gently:** Use gentle, reassuring non-verbal communication and maintain a calm demeanor to avoid emotional upset.
- **Focus on Providing Physical Support:** Offer assistance with eating, bathing, toileting, and any other daily activities that require physical effort.
- **Consider Extra Support:** Should you need more help, professional caregiving or residential care options are available and may be an option.
- **Plan for Transitional Care:** Review or establish a plan for end-of-life care. Update medical documents, as needed. Make sure final arrangements are in place.

The Power of Preparation

Understanding the usual progression of Alzheimer's dementia and knowing what to expect at each stage can help caregivers prepare and provide the most effective support to a person living with Alzheimer's. Each stage presents unique challenges, but with knowledge, support, and resources, caregivers can navigate this journey with compassion and resilience.

Section Two
Care Strategies for Each Stage

Kim was sitting across from her dad, sharing a light-hearted moment over morning coffee, when suddenly he couldn't recall a common word—a word he had used easily a thousand times before. There was a brief flicker of confusion in his eyes, quickly veiled. Looking back, Kim realized it was subtle moments like these, which she often dismissed as mere slips of the mind, that were signaling the onset of early stage Alzheimer's.

Learning to recognize, understand, and adapt to the changing needs of your loved one, is one of the most important skills you'll develop as a caregiver.

In this section, we'll discuss how Alzheimer's care needs to adapt during each stage of the disease. From setting up routines and safety measures in the early stages, managing sudden behavioral changes and physical symptoms in the middle stages, to focusing on quality of life in the late stages, each phase requires specific strategies to meet the evolving needs of your loved one.

Early Stage Alzheimer's Care

In the early stages of Alzheimer's, the changes can be very subtle and are often mistaken for normal aging or simple stress. This phase can be particularly challenging because it's about recognizing the unknown and catching those small signs before they become more obvious. During stages one to three of Alzheimer's, your loved one might still enjoy hobbies, social activities, and managing their daily routines. They may seem perfectly normal in social settings, keeping their condition hidden from others. It's usually in the more intimate settings of home where you might start noticing subtle shifts.

The first signs can be as simple as forgetting familiar names or misplacing household items, which could easily be shrugged off by anyone. But then, more telling symptoms may appear, like difficulty in performing tasks that require planning or problem-solving, challenges in completing familiar tasks at home or work, or trouble with words when speaking or writing. It's not just about forgetfulness; it might also show up as mood changes or even withdrawal from social activities they once enjoyed. These changes are often gradual, making them easy to miss unless you're looking closely.

These early signs are indicators you'll want to understand. They call for a proactive approach to managing Alzheimer's, focusing not just on medication or treatment but on maintaining a rich and fulfilling life. The goal at this stage is to slow the progression, cushion the impact on daily life, and, most importantly, adapt your support to meet the changing needs of your loved one. This might involve setting up simple reminders around the house, organizing their space more efficiently, or finding gentle ways to assist with tasks without taking over, thus preserving their sense of independence and dignity.

One of the most empowering things you can do at this stage is to educate yourself about the disease. Understanding Alzheimer's prepares you for the practical aspects of caregiving and equips you to handle the emotional challenges that come with it. It helps you recognize that their frustration or withdrawal isn't personal; it's part of the disease. With this knowledge, your approach can shift from a place of correction or frustration to one of compassion and patience.

In these early stages, your role is like that of a gentle guide. You're there to support and assist, helping to clear the fog that Alzheimer's brings. It's about making the home a sanctuary where confusion is met with calmness, changes are handled with care, and your loved one feels safe and supported. This stage is about ensuring legal and financial documents are in place, and laying a foundation of routines and safety measures that can evolve as the disease progresses. This ensures that as challenges grow, so does your ability to handle them gracefully and effectively.

Navigating early stage Alzheimer's involves practical adjustments in daily living and finding ways to maintain emotional connections. It's about finding those moments of clarity and connection, cherishing them, and using them as a reminder of the person behind the disease.

Remember that every effort you make on this journey shows your strength and dedication, leading to a deeper understanding of Alzheimer's and speaking to the remarkable resilience of the human spirit.

Initiating a Structured Routine

Creating a consistent daily routine for someone with early stage Alzheimer's is like setting the stage for a smoother day, every day. Think of a routine as a gentle framework that supports your loved one, reducing the chaos that cognitive decline can bring. In these early stages, they might still have a good grip on many aspects of their daily life, but confusion and forgetfulness can start to cause stress and anxiety. A predictable routine helps reduce these uncertainties, providing a comforting structure that makes everything a little less confusing.

When Jasper's father, Sam, was diagnosed with early stage Alzheimer's, Jasper wanted to help him feel secure and less anxious. Remembering how much Sam loved creating artwork, Jasper set up a small art studio in the garage. Every morning after breakfast, they spent an hour together working in the studio. Afterward, they'd take a walk around the neighborhood, enjoying the fresh air and getting some light exercise. Lunch was followed by a short nap to keep Sam rested and calm. In the afternoons, they'd do some light gardening or stretches. This routine made Sam's days more predictable, and provided Sam with a sense of peace.

Routine is powerful; it creates a rhythm that can guide a person with Alzheimer's through their day with more confidence. When activities happen at the same time each day—meals, medication times, physical activity, and bedtime—they require less cognitive effort to manage.

This not only conserves your loved one's mental energy but also reduces the anxiety that unpredictability may cause. Maintaining these routines also helps manage the progression of Alzheimer's symptoms. As the condition evolves, you can slowly adjust established routines, which is often less jarring than sudden changes.

Creating a daily schedule might seem daunting at first, but approaching it incrementally can help it feel less overwhelming. Start by aligning key activities with the natural rhythms of the day. For instance, schedule meals, medications, and bedtime at the same times each day to create reliable anchors for your loved one. Make sure there's enough time for rest to prevent fatigue, which can worsen confusion and irritability. Tailor physical activity to their current ability level; even light exercise like a walk in the park, walking the dog, or simple stretching can significantly boost mood and overall health. Remember, the goal isn't just to structure their day but to balance activity with adequate rest, ensuring they don't feel overwhelmed.

Incorporating activities that your loved one enjoys and can perform independently is vital. Engaging in hobbies or interests they have always enjoyed can provide a sense of normalcy and pleasure. For someone who's an avid reader, this might mean setting aside time each day to flip through a novel or listen to an audiobook. For someone who is an artist, it could mean drawing cartoons on blank sheets of paper, coloring in coloring books, or painting on canvas. These activities are not just ways to pass time; they are vital for maintaining cognitive function, emotional health, and motor skills. They stimulate the mind and help keep your loved one engaged with the world around them.

Change is inevitable, especially as Alzheimer's progresses, and adapting the routine to accommodate these changes is important. Introduce changes gradually to avoid overwhelming your loved one.

If a new medication needs to be integrated into the daily regimen or a physical therapy session needs to be scheduled, try to introduce these changes one at a time. Communication plays a key role here; talk through any changes with your loved one, explaining why they are necessary and how they will fit into the day. This helps ease the transition and involves them in their own care, increasing their cooperation and making the adjustment smoother.

It's important to establish a routine with regular times for critical tasks. Add enjoyable and stimulating activities, and handle changes thoughtfully to create a supportive daily structure. This improves both their quality of life and yours, making the path you walk together a bit easier to navigate.

Creating a Safe Home

As a caregiver, making the home a safe, comforting sanctuary can do wonders for both you and your loved one. Here, we'll go over practical ways to modify your home to meet their evolving needs, ensure their safety, and improve their quality of life.

> *When Sally first started adjusting her home for her mother, she discovered something new every day—rugs that were tripping hazards, a bathroom that needed more accessible features, and kitchen appliances that posed risks. Addressing these issues not only reduced the chances of accidents but also helped her mother maintain her independence a little bit longer.*

Begin by walking through your home at different times of the day to spot potential safety hazards that might not be obvious at first. Look for loose carpets that could slip, dim lighting that might obscure obstacles, or furniture that gets in the way of walking. Making a checklist during your walk-through can help you address each area of your home and make sure nothing is overlooked.

Next, start by making modifications. In the bathroom, installing grab bars by the toilet and in the shower can prevent falls, while a shower seat and a hand-held shower head can make bathing easier and safer. In the kitchen, securing rugs with non-slip pads and installing automatic shut-off devices on the stove and faucets can help prevent accidents. If stairs are a concern, setting up gates at the top and bottom can prevent unsupervised access. Clearly marking the steps with high-contrast tape can also be useful for someone whose vision and perception might be declining.

Creating a calming environment is just as important as looking out for someone's physical safety. Alzheimer's can make it difficult to process a lot of sensory input, leading to confusion and anxiety. To create a more calming space, paint the walls with soothing colors like blue and green, reduce clutter to minimize overstimulation, and control noise levels in your home.

Lighting plays a big role too. Make sure that your home is well-lit to reduce shadows and glare, which can be disorienting. Consider using bulbs that mimic natural light to help maintain circadian rhythms and support better sleep patterns. Automated lighting systems that turn on when someone gets out of bed at night can prevent falls and provide a sense of security.

Surveillance systems like cameras and audio monitors help you keep an eye on your loved one while respecting their dignity and privacy. Strategically placed cameras can monitor their activities without being intrusive, helping to keep them safe when alone in a room or during the night. It's essential to discuss with family members the extent and purpose of monitoring to respect ethical considerations.

Devices worn as pendants or wristbands with buttons to call for help, often including fall detection technology, can be invaluable. These devices signal for help automatically if a fall is detected, even if the person doesn't press the button. This helps your loved one maintain a sense of independence and improves safety outcomes as well.

Finally, make sure you're prepared for a potential emergency. Set up a clearly marked and easily accessible emergency kit that contains medical information, extra medication, and emergency contact numbers. Regularly update this kit and review its contents with other family members. Conduct drills to practice what to do in case of an emergency, so that everyone knows how to respond quickly and safely. Maintaining open lines of communication with neighbors and local Alzheimer's associations can also provide extra support and quick assistance when needed.

By taking these steps, you not only safeguard the physical well-being of your loved one, but also contribute to a more stable and reassuring atmosphere. This proactive approach improves the quality of life for your loved one and provides peace of mind for everyone involved in their care.

Tackling Nutritional Challenges

Alzheimer's can significantly impact a person's ability to eat and absorb food properly, leading to several challenges that you, as a caregiver, must be able to manage proactively.

One common issue is a decreased appetite, which can cause your loved one to show less interest in food or even skip meals altogether. This can happen for a variety of reasons, such as changes in taste preferences, dental problems, or a decreased sense of smell and taste. Forgetfulness can also be a big factor; your loved one might simply forget to eat or think they have already eaten. These eating challenges pose significant nutritional risks. Weight loss is a frequent concern and can lead to fatigue, muscle weakness, and a compromised immune system.

> *Kevin had always considered himself to be about 10 pounds overweight. As he approached the middle stages of Alzheimer's, he would often forget to eat. Within a matter of months, he had lost over 40 pounds and appeared unusually thin. Kevin didn't notice the weight loss until his family and friends expressed concern. His family then implemented special dietary routines to ensure he received the necessary nutrition. Although he never regained the lost weight, his weight did stabilize.*

Hydration is another necessary, yet often overlooked, aspect of nutrition. People with Alzheimer's might forget to drink enough fluids, or they may not feel thirsty, leading to dehydration. Dehydration can lead to urinary tract infections, constipation, and even more severe complications like kidney problems. Making sure your loved one drinks enough throughout the day is imperative. Keep water easily accessible, encourage them to take regular sips, and provide beverages that you know they enjoy. Using clear cups can help them see what's inside, making it more likely they'll drink. Incorporating foods with high water content like cucumbers, watermelons, and oranges can also help them stay hydrated.

Making sure that your loved one receives a balanced diet is important and can make a huge difference in managing their condition. A diet that supports brain health and overall well-being should include a variety of nutrients. For example, omega-3 fatty acids, found in fish like salmon and seeds like flax seeds, are essential for brain health and have anti-inflammatory properties. Antioxidants, which help protect brain cells from damage, are abundant in fruits and vegetables like berries and spinach. Vitamins E and C, as well as B vitamins, play key roles in cognitive health and nervous system support. These vitamins can be found in nuts, citrus fruits, and whole grains. Nutrient deficiencies from reduced food intake can affect everything from skin health to cognitive function. Adding these nutrients to your loved one's diet can help manage symptoms and possibly slow cognitive decline.

Tips for Managing Medications

Properly managing medications is crucial when caring for someone with Alzheimer's. The right medications can manage unwanted symptoms and greatly improve your loved one's quality of life. However, this process doesn't always come without challenges. In the hopes of setting you up for success in this area, here are some steps you can use to ease your mind and allow you to stay on top of everything related to medication:

1. **Establish a Consistent Routine:** Having your loved one take their medication at the same time everyday can help them remember to take it. If you can, try to get them to associate different medications to different activities, like eating breakfast or brushing their teeth before bed.

2. **Use Pill Organizers:** Finding an error-proof system for organizing medications is key. It can be too easy for someone with Alzheimer's to accidentally skip a dose or take a pill more often than they're supposed to. Investing in pill organizers that are marked with days of the week and times of day helps ensure the right dose is taken at the correct time while letting you easily check whether any doses have been missed.

3. **Incorporate Technology:** Setting alarms on a smartphone or using an app to remind you when medications need to be taken can help your loved one stay on track while also

keeping you in the loop. This is especially true when memory is an issue.

4. **Communicate Openly:** It's natural for someone with Alzheimer's to be skeptical of taking medications, and resistance can be expected. Sometimes your loved one might feel overwhelmed by the number of pills or believe they don't have a need for them. It's important to clearly communicate the purpose of each pill in simple terms and reinforce how it benefits their health.

5. **Make Adjustments As Needed:** Note any changes in symptoms or side effects. Regularly review the medication regimen with a healthcare provider to adjust dosages or change prescriptions for continued effectiveness.

6. **Keep Track of Side Effects:** Side effects are often a reality of medication use, but proactively managing them can prevent further complications. Note side effects like nausea, dizziness, or changes in appetite, which can all affect quality of life. Be prepared to discuss these with a doctor. If certain side effects become problematic, the healthcare provider might adjust the medications to help your loved one be more comfortable.

7. **Ensure Compliance:** If forgetfulness becomes a regular occurrence, your loved one may need additional reminders or more supervision. In cases where your loved one is resistant to taking medication, reassess the need for each medication with your healthcare provider; it might be possible to simplify the regimen to make it less overwhelming for both of you.

Medication Dispensers

Dispensing medications accurately and consistently can be tricky, but there are several dispensers available beyond the standard plastic trays and cups labeled SUN-SAT and AM or PM.

- **Round Automatic Pill Dispensers:** These battery-operated devices can hold up to 28 days of medications, depending on the dosage frequency. They rotate to the next dose on schedule, helping your loved one take their medication at the correct times.
- **AC-Powered Pill Dispensers:** These dispensers often have advanced computer technology and are more secure. Some provide caregiver notifications and can hold at least a 90-day supply of medications. They help maintain independence in the early and middle stages of Alzheimer's and assist caregivers in the later stages as well.

My mother wanted the autonomy to manage her own medications, but she was finding it increasingly difficult to do so. We tried several medication dispensers, but they were either too difficult for her to retrieve the meds, or too difficult for her to know for certain that she had taken the right meds at the right time.

The MedaCube™ (sold only in the U.S. and Canada) was my personal choice for managing my mother's medications. The device verbally reminded her when it was time to take her meds, how to retrieve them, and to close the drawer when she was done. I loved it because it was distraction-free. Since she couldn't see her medication supply, she didn't try to move the meds around. I was also able to record my voice to describe each medication, which served as a helpful and comforting guide for my mother. We both fell in love with the machine because we felt confident that she was getting the correct medications at the right time. I also got a text message if meds were not taken, or the supply was running low. Plus, I was finally able to take a vacation without worrying about managing medications!

Building a Caregiving Team

If you've ever tried juggling multiple responsibilities alone, then you know it's both challenging and not sustainable. This is especially true when caring for someone with Alzheimer's, where the demands can be both challenging and ever-changing. Establishing a caregiving team is not just helpful, but necessary. The truth is, going at it alone can lead to burnout, decreased quality of care, and poor health. Having a group of trusted individuals to share responsibilities with can greatly alleviate your stress and improve the quality of care you provide.

A well-rounded caregiving team can include family members, friends, professional caregivers, and healthcare professionals, each bringing their own strengths and expertise to the table. This collaborative approach covers all aspects of care, including daily personal care, medical management, and emotional support.

Initially, when the symptoms of Alzheimer's are milder, the team might be smaller. Perhaps you manage day-to-day care with occasional help from family and periodic check-ins with medical professionals. However, as the disease progresses, you'll likely need a more robust team, including professional caregivers or home health aides to handle the increasing demands.

Without a team, pressure can mount on a single caregiver, creating overwhelm and leading to physical and emotional exhaustion. Having to be "on" 24/7 without a break is challenging for anyone and can lead to feelings of isolation, resentment, and even depression. It's hard for one person to have to manage everything, from complex medication schedules to legal and financial planning. This is why having a team where tasks are shared based on each person's skills and availability is so important.

As Alzheimer's progresses, the roles within your caregiving team will naturally change. Initially, the focus may be on companionship and support with daily tasks. However, as the disease advances, caregiving will become more complex, requiring additional medical and safety expertise. Regularly reassessing the team's structure will help meet the evolving needs of your loved one.

> *Maria lived alone, with no family close by. When she was diagnosed with Alzheimer's, she shared this information with her best friend, Robinetta, who was a retired nurse and who had already been designated as her Medical Decision Maker. Together, they decided that Maria would bring in a part time caregiver for the early stages, who could eventually become a full time caregiver. This would give Maria time to get to know and trust having a new person in her home. She also decided to have her Power of Attorney for Finances partner with her to start managing her finances immediately. In speaking with the family, there was a cousin who was happy to exchange room and board for caregiving and a small stipend through the middle and late stages, so that a second full time caregiver would not need to be hired. The family understood that Robinetta would oversee medical decisions, handle in-home care as needed, and provide regular family updates. This initial plan lowered Maria's anxiety. It also helped Robinetta and the family feel supported as they worked together as a team to provide for the variety of caregiving needs.*

Building and maintaining a caregiving team requires open communication and flexibility. Regular meetings or updates help keep everyone on the same page and allow for adjustments to care plans as needed. These gatherings are also a time to address any conflicts or challenges and make sure the team works well together. Remember, each member of the team, including you, needs support and occasional respite to sustain the compassion and energy required for this role.

By sharing the responsibilities of caregiving, you not only increase the amount of support your loved one has, but also build a community of care that extends beyond the confines of immediate family. This network can be a tremendous source of emotional comfort and practical help as you navigate the complexities of Alzheimer's together. Through teamwork, you provide your loved one with the best possible support throughout all stages of their condition, allowing you to cherish more good days together, even amidst the challenges.

Roles and Responsibilities in a Caregiving Team

Building a caregiving team is all about finding the right person for each role. This process is much like building a house, where every member of the team acts as a different part of the structure. From the foundation to the walls to the roof, each person provides valuable support to ensure safety and stability.

When thinking about potential team members from your family members, friends, and greater community, consider not just their willingness to help but also their suitability based on their strengths, weaknesses, and availability. This initial step involves recognizing who can contribute what, balancing emotional closeness with practical skills. For instance, a friend who is a nurse or has medical training might be perfect for managing health care tasks, while a retired neighbor could help with daily chores or provide companionship. It's about making use of everyone's unique strengths to benefit the whole group while also making sure no one is overworked.

Approaching potential team members requires sensitivity and clear communication. Start by thoroughly explaining the situation—discuss the nature of Alzheimer's, the specific needs of your loved one, and the kind of help you're looking for. Be honest about the challenges but also highlight the rewarding aspects of being part of a caregiving team. It's important to give potential members a realistic picture so they can make an informed decision about their involvement. Remember, the goal here is not just to fill roles but to create a supportive network that works well together for the benefit of your loved one.

Once you have volunteers, assign roles based on their skills, preferences, and availability. This personalized approach helps each team member feel capable and confident in their responsibilities, greatly improving the overall effectiveness and harmony of the group.

Setting clear expectations and boundaries is essential. This includes defining each person's responsibilities and agreeing on ways to communicate and resolve conflicts. Regular check-ins are helpful for discussing what's working and what isn't, and making necessary adjustments to roles and tasks. These meetings also give everyone a chance to acknowledge one another's contributions, which can reinforce a sense of team unity and purpose. Clear boundaries help prevent misunderstandings and respect each team member's personal limits, which supports their ongoing commitment.

Regular team meetings are key to staying coordinated and adapting to the changing needs of your loved one. These meetings should be scheduled at times that make sense based on the progression of the disease and team dynamics, but more frequent meetings might be necessary as the disease advances. During these meetings, discuss updates on your loved one's condition, any changes in medication or treatment plans, and adjustments in caregiving responsibilities. This is also an opportunity to share feelings and experiences, which can be therapeutic and help strengthen the support network. To ensure these meetings are productive, prepare an agenda, take notes, and consider rotating who leads each time.

This balanced approach to building and managing a caregiving team makes the most of everyone's strengths while providing the emotional and practical support needed to address the challenges of Alzheimer's care. By taking advantage of each team member's unique abilities, you can build a resilient support system that meets the needs of your loved one and supports one another along the way.

Navigating Family Discussions and Dynamics in Alzheimer's Care

When caring for a loved one with Alzheimer's, family dynamics play an integral role in both the quality of care provided and the emotional health of everyone involved. Open and honest communication is the foundation of effective caregiving, and approaching these conversations can sometimes feel as complex as managing the medical aspects of Alzheimer's itself. Creating an environment where every family member feels heard, valued, and informed is key to fostering a cooperative and supportive environment.

Start by making sure everyone understands the realities of Alzheimer's disease—its progression, the care required, and the emotional toll it may take. Planning a family meeting can be an effective and heartfelt way to share this information and discuss how to move forward as a unit. When organizing the meeting, choose a time and place where everyone feels comfortable and won't be distracted. Making and sharing a list of topics to be covered beforehand helps keep the meeting on track and allows everyone to prepare questions and express their thoughts and feelings.

During the meeting, use clear and gentle language. Consider using visual aids like diagrams or short videos to explain more complex issues, such as the stages of Alzheimer's or how it affects the brain. These tools can make these topics easier to understand, especially for family members who may not have a medical background. Encourage questions and be ready to address common concerns, which can range from daily care routines to the financial implications of long-term care. Respond with empathy, recognizing that many questions stem from fear, frustration, or grief.

Setting expectations is another fundamental part of these discussions. Be honest about the challenges ahead and what will likely be required in terms of time, effort, and emotional investment. It's equally important to talk about the potential roles each family member might play. These roles should be assigned not just based on schedules or proximity but also on emotional capacity and personal strengths. For example, someone who can't help with day-to-day care might take on administrative tasks like managing medical appointments or financial planning.

Balancing these roles is key to preventing caregiver burnout and making sure no one feels overwhelmed or underutilized. Regular check-ins can help your family adjust roles as needed and provide ongoing support for primary caregivers who might bear the brunt of daily caregiving responsibilities. It can also be helpful to engage distant family members who might want to contribute but are unsure how. Simple efforts like regularly scheduled video calls can allow them to stay connected and involved.

Conflicts will inevitably arise, often centered around differing opinions on care decisions or the distribution of responsibilities. When these occur, focus on finding collaborative solutions that prioritize the well-being of your loved one with Alzheimer's. Techniques like active listening, where each person's concerns are fully heard before responding, can be incredibly effective. Sometimes, bringing in an impartial mediator, such as a counselor or a professional familiar with caregiving dynamics, can help resolve more entrenched conflicts by providing fresh perspectives and encouraging understanding among family members.

Supporting younger family members through this process is also imperative. Children and teenagers might struggle to understand what's happening or express their feelings about the changes they see in their loved one. Explaining Alzheimer's in age-appropriate terms and involving them in smaller caregiving responsibilities can help them feel connected and less afraid. Open conversations about their feelings and fears can help them manage this challenging time.

Handling family dynamics effectively requires patience, planning, and a lot of heart. It's about making sure everyone is on the same page, feels supported, and is able to contribute to the collective goal of providing the best possible care for your loved one with Alzheimer's. By fostering open communication, setting clear expectations, and managing conflicts with empathy and understanding, you strengthen not only the network of support around your loved one but also the bonds within your family.

Communicating Effectively with Healthcare Professionals

Navigating the healthcare system and communicating with medical professionals can feel overwhelming, especially when you're advocating for someone with Alzheimer's. However, developing a solid communication plan can help your loved one receive the best care possible.

Start by compiling a list of all healthcare providers involved in their care, including their specialties, contact information, and the best times to reach them. This directory will be your go-to resource for managing appointments, understanding treatment plans, and addressing any emergencies.

Preparing for medical appointments is another area to pay close attention to. Keep an up-to-date summary of your loved one's medical history, current medications, and any recent changes in their health or behavior. This document should be concise yet comprehensive, providing a quick snapshot for healthcare providers who may not be familiar with your loved one's medical history. Before each appointment, write down a list of questions or concerns you have, prioritizing them from most to least urgent. This ensures that you cover all critical points during the consultation.

Understanding medical terminology can be daunting, but familiarizing yourself with some common terms used in Alzheimer's care can greatly increase your confidence and ability to make informed decisions. There are many resources available, from online medical dictionaries to pamphlets and books designed for caregivers. Don't be afraid to ask healthcare providers to explain terms and concepts if something isn't clear. This new knowledge can help you understand your loved one better and communicate more effectively with their medical team.

Technology can also be a useful ally. Many healthcare systems now offer patient portals, which allow you to access medical records, schedule appointments, and communicate directly with doctors. These tools make it easier to keep track of appointments, test results, and treatment updates. Be sure to have your loved one provide you with access to their medical records in these systems. Telemedicine services are also beneficial for caregivers who find it challenging to attend in-person appointments due to responsibilities or mobility concerns.

By building a strong communication foundation, thoroughly preparing for appointments, understanding medical terms, and using technology, you can make your interactions with healthcare professionals more effective and productive. This proactive approach not only helps manage the medical aspects of Alzheimer's care but also provides peace of mind, reminding you that you're doing everything in your power to advocate for and support your loved one.

Early Stage Communication Techniques

Having conversations with someone in the early stages of Alzheimer's requires a gentle touch, patience, and a few adjustments to how we typically communicate.

Active listening is key when talking with a person who has Alzheimer's. This means truly listening to what they're trying to express, both verbally and non-verbally. It involves giving them your full attention, nodding, and responding in ways that show you're engaged and understanding.

Recognizing and acknowledging their feelings is essential, even if what they say doesn't entirely make sense. If they express a worry that seems misplaced, rather than correcting them, validate their feelings by saying something like, "This sounds like something that's really bothering you. I'm here for you, and we can figure it out together." This approach shows you care about their emotions and helps maintain your connection.

Non-verbal communication often speaks louder than words, especially when verbal skills start to wane. Your body language, facial expressions, and tone of voice can convey empathy, patience, and understanding. A gentle touch on the arm, a warm smile, or a calm, soothing tone can provide reassurance and comfort, often more effectively than words could.

Being mindful of your loved one's non-verbal cues can also be pivotal in understanding their needs and feelings, even when they might struggle to express themselves verbally. For instance, if they seem distressed or uncomfortable, they might not be able to articulate it directly, but their body language—such as fidgeting or looking away —can give you clues about how they're feeling.

Knowing how to handle communication breakdowns gracefully is critical. There will be moments of misunderstanding or frustration as the disease affects your loved one's ability to communicate. Staying patient during these times is key. If a conversation becomes too challenging, light humor can help ease tension, but ensure it's not at their expense and that it's understood and appreciated. Sometimes, taking a short break and revisiting the conversation later can help both of you reset and approach the interaction with renewed patience.

When communicating with someone in the early stages of Alzheimer's, your goal is to foster understanding and maintain a loving connection. It's about adapting to their needs, listening deeply, and responding with kindness and patience. Through thoughtful communication strategies, you can address the complexities of Alzheimer's, helping your loved one feel supported and valued every step of the way.

Establishing Essential Planning Documents

Approaching a conversation about end-of-life care with a person who has Alzheimer's can be incredibly difficult. You might worry about upsetting them or wonder if it's the right time. Having these discussions early, while your loved one can still express their wishes and participate in decisions, is crucial. It ensures their preferences are understood and respected when they might no longer be able to communicate them.

To start, choose a time when you both feel relaxed and not rushed, like after a meal or during a slow afternoon. Choose a comfortable place free from distractions. Approach the topic with sensitivity and openness, emphasizing the importance of honoring their wishes and providing the care they desire at each stage. Be patient, as these conversations may take several weeks to complete.

There are three main themes you will want to cover during these conversations:

1. How care and support are provided now and through the middle stages
2. How care is provided during the late stages
3. Decisions about what to do at the time of death and afterward

Opening Discussion - Planning Documents

Start by talking about what medical, legal, and insurance documents are already in place. Consider the list below and ask if there are any more documents you should know about. Note which ones are missing so you can address them later. (Refer to the Legal and Financial Planning section of this book for more details.)

- **Durable Power of Attorney for Healthcare (DPOA for Healthcare or Medical Decision Maker)**
- **Financial Durable Power of Attorney (DPOA for Finances)**
- **Trust or Will**
- **Long Term Care Insurance**
- **POLST**
- **Final Arrangements:** Many people have paid for these final arrangements in advance because they have family plots, put this information in a Will/Trust, or feel strongly about what happens to their body after they die.

Discussion for Early to Middle Stages Care - Planning Documents

Encourage your loved one to review, update, and/or establish whatever planning documents are not yet completed. It is helpful for your loved one to decide on the kind of support they want during the early to middle stages. This includes confirming legal decision-makers for health and finances as well as considering additional support needs.

- **Healthcare DPOA:** Make sure the names and contact information for the designated medical decision maker and any backups are documented and kept current. Confirm that these individuals are aware of their role, agree to it, and have copies of all necessary documents. Your loved one might want to update the document to activate the decision maker's role immediately, involving them in medical appointments. This allows the medical team to become familiar with the decision maker and will make things easier later.
- **Financial DPOA:** Review or establish this document, verify that all information is accurate, and confirm that the appointed person agrees to the role and has up-to-date contact details. It's important for your loved one to start "training" this person on managing their finances. Once your loved one can no longer remember all their financial matters, it may take a while to figure everything out and get necessary access. Subtle things may be missed without their realization.

John had his way of managing the family finances and never wanted any interference from anyone. As he started realizing that simple math was becoming more difficult, however, he spoke with his wife and they agreed to have their son, Ted, start taking over managing their finances. John updated his DPOA for finances document to allow Ted's role to be immediately effective, without giving up his rights to make decisions as well. John accompanied Ted to the banks and other financial institutions to file the DPOA paperwork, to make things easier for Ted, as John was still able to make his own decisions. One banker explained that if John had waited until he could not accompany Ted, Ted would have needed to get a doctor's note in addition to the DPOA paperwork to set up Ted's privileges. As John and Ted partnered on managing the household finances, Ted discovered the life insurance policy was a couple of months late. Ted was able to bring the account current before it was canceled. John was so relieved to learn that his wife would still have the life insurance available when he died, because he'd never qualify for a policy like that now.

As your loved one progresses through Alzheimer's, they will need more support. Review financial resources to discuss when, and if, additional household support can be added, like housekeepers, personal assistants, or aides who can help with driving, light housekeeping, and meal prep. Sometimes this additional person is a family member, and the home may need to be adjusted for this caregiver to have a room to sleep in at night.

Here are some other reminders for this stage:

- Discuss any other support your loved one might need. Deepen the conversation by really getting to know what gives life meaning and joy for them.
- Discuss what music they like listening to, or books they like to read.
- What are their hobbies and pastimes?

- Note who they enjoy visiting and having come over to visit. Who do they not want to see?
- What are their dietary and menu preferences?
- What makes them feel calm, relaxed, and peaceful?
- What are their spiritual preferences and how do they want to live those preferences out?
- What is most important to them to maintain their privacy and dignity?

Discussion for Late Stage Care - Ensuring Quality of Life

Understanding your loved one's wishes during their final journey through Alzheimer's will help you honor them when the time comes. Some family members feel guilty at this stage because they don't know what their loved one wants or don't have the finances to honor their wishes. Here are some steps you can take to alleviate those guilty feelings and make sure your loved one's wishes are honored:

- **Discuss Pain Management:** Determine how your loved one feels about pain and pain medication, including opioids. This conversation might require follow-up with a medical professional to clarify any misconceptions and address fears for both of you.
- **Determine Future Living Arrangements:** Discuss and decide how to recognize when your loved one is ready to move to an assisted living facility or memory care unit. Understand the costs involved for these services in your area and plan how you'll manage these finances. Consulting with an accountant may be necessary to prepare financially.
- **Plan for Home Care:** If care is provided in the home, what will the caregiving team look like? This is not a one-person job. Will there be private caregivers, or will the family rotate support?

- **Honor Spiritual or Faith Traditions:** What spiritual or faith traditions need to be honored as the Alzheimer's journey continues? Who needs to be notified or invited to visit to provide spiritual or religious support? For example, if your loved one goes out for lunch with a close group of friends once a month, how can that be maintained over time? How might you transition that from visits out, to visits in the home, to video and telephone calls over time? What religious leaders would your loved one like to be invited during the journey to provide faith based support, or end of life support?

Discussion on Final Arrangements - What Happens After Death

Talking about life after death can be a difficult topic or an easy one. Some people are very clear on how they want to die and what they want to be done with their remains. Others will refuse to have this discussion and leave it up to you. Many will be grateful you raised the topic instead of attempting to guess at their wishes.

If final arrangements have been made, locate the documents and verify the information. Some final arrangement details to discuss and keep in mind include:

- **Mortuary/Funeral Home:** These are the people who will pick up your loved one's body and prepare it for the next steps. If you have hospice care at home or your loved one is in a facility, you will be asked to provide this information as soon as possible after admission.
- **What happens to the body?** Options include burial, cremation, or donation to science. Non-traditional methods like green burial and human composting are also

available. Cremated remains have even more novel choices, like being turned into diamonds, launched into space, or turned into fireworks. If your loved one doesn't care, note that direct cremation may be the least expensive method. Burial averages $12K-30K, while cremation is usually $1K - $2K. If your loved one has the funds, encourage them to pay for these arrangements now, as prices may increase significantly in the future.

- **Memorials and Funerals:** What does your loved one want? Some people expect a funeral or memorial at their place of worship. Others want a private memorial, a graveside service, or their ashes scattered at sea. Knowing these wishes helps you honor your loved one after they are gone.

When Tom was diagnosed with Alzheimer's, he took the time to share his final wishes with his family. He wanted his ashes to be buried on their family land, with a tree planted on top as a living tribute to his life. His family found solace in this meaningful request. After Tom passed away, they made sure to fulfill his wish. Each year, they visit the tree, which now stands tall and strong, as a reminder of Tom's spirit. The tree has become a special place for them to remember him, reflecting his love for his family and the powerful legacy left behind.

Some people with Alzheimer's may initially not want to have these discussions at all and leave all the decisions to their family. Honor your culture and family traditions, recognizing that these discussions can stir deep emotions. Sometimes, you'll need to revisit certain conversations as things change during your caregiving journey.

Finally, organize a family meeting to review your loved one's decisions. Update any necessary documents and address all questions. It's imperative to have this discussion while your loved one can still participate, ensuring that their wishes are clearly understood and allowing the family to feel more confident in the care plan as it is put into action.

This thoughtful approach ensures that when faced with difficult decisions, you're guided not only by medical considerations but also by a deep respect for your loved one's expressed wishes and personal dignity.

Middle Stage Alzheimer's Care

As familiar aspects of their personality shift and their independence decreases, your role as a caregiver becomes more challenging and more important. Adapting your strategies to cope with these changes is critical. Here, we'll talk about what you might be able to expect during this period and how you can best support your loved one through these transitions.

In the middle stages of Alzheimer's, typically covering stages four and five, cognitive decline becomes more pronounced. This is when the symptoms of the disease become more evident and start to interfere significantly with daily life. You might notice your loved one becoming more forgetful of recent events or personal details that were previously familiar. They may start having difficulties with spatial awareness or language, sometimes struggling to recall the right word or name. You may also begin to see changes in their behavior that can be unexpected and, at times, distressing.

One of the most heart-wrenching behaviors is wandering, which can be both confusing and dangerous if not managed properly. You might find that your loved one begins to walk aimlessly, often driven by an unclear desire or confusion about their surroundings.

Another common issue is sundowning—increased confusion and agitation that occur in the late afternoon and evening. These behaviors are challenging for your loved one and can be exhausting and worrying for you as a caregiver.

You may also notice uncharacteristic behaviors such as hoarding, increased agitation, or becoming more easily upset. Aggression, hallucinations, and even paranoia can appear during these stages, which can be particularly difficult to manage. These behaviors often stem from frustration, fear, or confusion as your loved one struggles to make sense of a world that no longer feels familiar.

As my mother lost an inch of her height with age, she could no longer reach the shelves above the refrigerator. Her way of making sense of what was a sudden change for her, was to declare that someone had replaced her fridge with a taller one. Initially, she was quite mad about this. The more the family argued with her, the angrier and more aggressive she became. What worked for us was to acknowledge her feelings of how upsetting it would be to have someone replace one's fridge without being asked, without arguing about what was true or not. Acknowledging and validating her feelings calmed her down, and then we were able to easily distract her by talking about something that gave her pleasure.

Working through these changes requires patience, understanding, and a willingness to adapt. By recognizing these signs and learning how to respond, you can help make this stage of Alzheimer's more manageable for both you and your loved one.

Managing the middle stages of Alzheimer's requires a mix of patience, understanding, proactive strategies, emotional support, and sometimes, professional help. Your approach will need to be flexible, evolving with the daily changes in your loved one's behavior and abilities. Adapting daily routines to meet their cognitive and behavioral changes, while keeping as much consistency as possible, can reduce confusion and agitation.

Navigating this phase demands a lot of empathy, a strong support network, and a wealth of knowledge and skills. Remember, you're not alone in this. There are communities, resources, and professionals who can offer guidance and support. As you adjust your care strategies, keep focusing on the love and respect that underpins the relationship you share with your loved one.

Implementing Safety Strategies for Wandering

When your loved one starts to wander, it can feel like you're trying to steer through uncharted waters, hoping to bring them back safely. Wandering is common in middle stage Alzheimer's and can be triggered by confusion, restlessness, or unmet needs like hunger or needing to use the bathroom. Recognizing these early signs is crucial. It's about understanding why they're wandering—whether they're looking for something or trying to meet a basic need. By staying alert to these cues, you can step in early and redirect their attention, potentially reducing wandering.

Start with some preventive measures to help manage wandering. Make sure their basic needs are consistently met. Regular meal times and easy access to snacks can prevent hunger-related wandering, while keeping a routine bathroom schedule can help reduce anxiety and restlessness.

A secure home is fundamental to safety, security, and peace of mind. Smart locks and alarms secure your home and give you peace of mind by alerting you if a door is unexpectedly opened. Use child-proof door locks, install gates at staircases, and put safety devices in potentially dangerous areas like the kitchen to alert you if your loved one tries to access them unsupervised. This not only keeps your loved one safe but also puts you at ease. If these safety devices cause agitation or aggression, approach the situation calmly. Acknowledge their frustration and offer to help them with whatever they need.

Technology can be a big help when it comes to managing wandering. Consider using GPS trackers and wearable devices that alert you if your loved one leaves a designated safe area. These can be worn as wristbands or pendants and are incredibly useful for keeping them safe, especially if they do manage to slip out of the house. Devices like the 'AngelSense GPS Tracker' can be attached to clothing and provide real-time tracking, so you always know where your loved one is. These devices often come with geofencing features, allowing you to set safe zones and receive alerts if your loved one wanders out of these areas. Wearable tech like the 'Fitbit' or Apple Watch can monitor not just location but also vital signs such as heart rate, providing a comprehensive view of their physical state throughout the day.

Motion sensors in and around your home can also alert you to unusual activity, allowing you to act quickly. These devices aren't just gadgets; they extend your reach as a caregiver, helping you protect your loved one even when you're not right by their side.

Having a rapid response plan is essential in case your loved one does end up wandering. Keep a recent picture of the person and a physical description, including what they're wearing, handy. If they do wander off, use GPS tracking devices to locate them and inform local authorities and neighbors right away. Community support can be a lifesaver, often making the difference between a quick recovery and a prolonged search.

Creating a safe wandering path can also help. If you have the space, secure an area where your loved one can walk around freely without any risk. This could be a fenced yard or a safe path around the house. Make sure this area is free from hazards like pools of water, tools, or toxic plants. This way, they can satisfy their need to move around in a safe environment without the danger of wandering off.

Being prepared for emergencies isn't just about reacting when something happens; it's about having a plan in place before anything goes wrong. Develop a response plan that includes informing neighbors, local Alzheimer's associations, and law enforcement about your loved one's tendency to wander. Teach them effective ways to communicate and guide your loved one back to safety. Keep an updated list of emergency contacts, medical information, and any other important details easily accessible. This preparation provides a structured plan for quickly and safely locating your loved one if they get lost, minimizing risks and maintaining their safety.

In managing wandering, a mix of vigilance, preparedness, and the right tools can help you provide a safe environment for your loved one while preserving their dignity and independence as much as possible.

Bathing and Dressing Simplified

As your loved one enters the latter part of the middle stage, their ability to manage personal tasks independently diminishes. Setting routines for bathing and dressing is very useful as this time can reduce stress for both of you.

Bathing is about more than just getting clean; it involves privacy, comfort, and physical safety concerns, along with your loved one's sense of dignity. To make this process less daunting, consider using tools like a shower chair or a handheld showerhead. These can make the bathing experience safer and more manageable, allowing your loved one to participate in their care as much as possible.

Before the bath, make sure the water is warm enough, as older adults often feel the cold more intensely. Soft, soothing lighting can also make the space feel more relaxing and less clinical. During the bath, keep the dialogue open by explaining each step before you proceed. Use calm and reassuring tones to help your loved one feel secure and respected.

Dressing can be another challenging area, but making the process simpler can help your loved one maintain a sense of normalcy and independence. Try to find clothes with simple fastenings, elastic waistbands, and Velcro to make dressing easier for someone with declining motor skills. Whenever possible, lay out two outfits and let your loved one choose what they'd like to wear. This simple choice can significantly boost their sense of autonomy and involvement in daily life. Organize their wardrobe to make these choices easy, with frequently used items easily accessible. Remember, the goal is to reduce complexity without taking away their agency.

Meal Planning Made Easy

Making foods easier to eat is another practical step that can make a big difference, especially as the disease progresses and chewing or swallowing becomes more difficult. Preparing softer foods, like cooked vegetables, stews, and smoothies, are nutritious and easier to consume. Cutting food into small, manageable pieces or offering finger foods can also help maintain your loved one's ability to eat on their own. Small sandwiches, cut fruits, and bite-sized proteins are other great choices. If regular food intake becomes a challenge, nutritional supplements can help ensure your loved one is getting enough calories and nutrients. Consult with a healthcare provider to make sure the chosen supplements won't interfere with any medications or medical conditions.

Understanding these nutritional challenges and putting thoughtful strategies in place can make a big difference for your loved one. This proactive approach not only supports their physical health but also improves their quality of life, helping them enjoy meals and stay as independent as possible. As always, the small adjustments you make can have a significant impact, offering comfort and care through the simple, everyday act of sharing a meal together.

Creating a well-thought-out meal plan for your loved one can be a key part of maintaining their health and making experiences involving food enjoyable. When planning meals for the week, consider your loved one's nutritional needs, personal preferences, and dietary restrictions. For instance, if your loved one enjoys fish, incorporate meals like baked salmon or tuna salad, which are not only rich in omega-3 fatty acids but also easier to chew.

A sample meal plan might look like this:

- **Breakfast:** Oatmeal with diced apples, cinnamon, and a sprinkle of flaxseed.
- **Lunch:** Chicken salad with lots of chopped veggies.
- **Dinner:** Soft stew with beef, potatoes, and carrots.

When preparing these meals, use cooking methods that preserve nutrients while making the food easy to eat. Steaming vegetables, for instance, retains more vitamins than boiling them, and baking fish with a drizzle of olive oil and herbs adds to its flavor without adding unnecessary fats. To make the food richer in flavor without adding excessive salt or sugar, use natural herbs and spices. Basil, rosemary, and turmeric not only boost flavor but also offer anti-inflammatory benefits, which are beneficial for cognitive health. Batch cooking, or meal prepping, can save you significant time by allowing you to prepare multiple servings of a dish at once. This approach provides ready meals for several days, easing the cooking process and helping maintain a consistent diet for your loved one.

For someone in the middle stages of Alzheimer's, being involved in the meal prep process can help them feel more engaged and independent. Depending on their abilities, they might be able to help with simple tasks like washing vegetables, stirring ingredients, or setting the table. These activities help them feel involved and also serve as cognitive exercises by keeping their mind engaged in familiar routines. To ensure safety in the kitchen, make sure to supervise your loved one and use adaptive kitchen tools designed to prevent injuries, such as knives with easy-grip handles or non-slip mats.

Finally, addressing common eating problems, such as loss of appetite or changed taste preferences, requires patience and creativity. If your loved one isn't hungry or they have a newfound preference for sweets, try making the flavor of their food better by using natural sweeteners like fruit or a small amount of honey instead of sugar. To manage portion sizes and regular calorie intake, try offering smaller, more frequent meals instead of three big meals per day.

Managing Hoarding and Mealtime Distractions

As Alzheimer's progresses, you might notice that your loved one may develop puzzling habits around food and mealtimes. They might forget when they last ate, which can lead to overeating or refusing to eat. This can result in nutritional imbalances or weight issues. Another common change is the tendency to hoard food, such as stashing snacks in odd places or insisting on keeping large quantities of certain foods on hand. This behavior often stems from anxiety or a fear of not having enough. Understanding this can help you approach the situation with empathy and patience.

To help manage these concerns, establish a regular routine for meals and snacks spaced evenly throughout the day. This can help stabilize blood sugar levels and reduce confusion about eating times, in addition to reducing the anxiety that drives hoarding. Use visual cues like a whiteboard or notepad to check off meals as they are eaten, serving as a reminder of their last mealtime. Gentle reminders of when they last ate, paired with a description of the meal, can also help orient them and reduce repeated eating or refusal to eat.

To help reduce hoarding, you can also create designated spaces in the kitchen, like a special shelf or a section in the refrigerator, where your loved one can store their "extra" food. This keeps the food safe and sanitary while respecting their need for control and security. Regularly check these spaces together to use or discard items, making this a shared activity that respects their independence and promotes safety.

> *Whenever Emily saw food that she liked, she would set aside a large quantity on a napkin or another plate. It soon became clear that her concern was that all the food would get eaten before she had enough. The family began to set a portion of the meal aside in the kitchen for her. They would reassure her regularly during the meal, that extra food was already set aside for her to eat later. After the meal, she was asked to put away the extra food that she wanted, that had been set aside for her. This stopped the hoarding during mealtime.*

Another common issue is distraction during meals. Your loved one may start eating but then get up to wander or lose focus, leaving the meal unfinished. This can make mealtime stressful and unsatisfying for both of you. To help keep your loved one focused, create a calm eating environment free from loud noises or visual distractions like a television. Engage them in light conversation about the food or other pleasant topics to keep their attention. If wandering is a concern, try scheduling meals at times when they are typically more settled, or use adaptive tableware designed to make eating easier and more engaging, such as plates with high contrast colors that differentiate food from the plate, making it easier to focus on the task of eating. Creating a calm eating environment free from distractions can help your loved one focus on their food and make mealtime a peaceful and enjoyable part of the day.

> *George often would get distracted during a meal. He would get up to change a fork and that would lead to one distraction after another. Sally would ask him to return to the table, and he'd keep saying, "I"m coming," and not return. Sally realized she had to engage George in choosing the dinnerware, and then during the meal, talk to him about the meal while providing gentle reminders to continue eating. This made George more comfortable during mealtimes and he eventually started finishing his meals.*

Handling these dietary related changes requires patience, creativity, and a willingness to adapt your strategies. By creating a structured yet flexible mealtime environment and addressing the underlying issues affecting their eating habits, you can help ensure that your loved one continues to enjoy meals and get the nutrition they need. The goal is to make mealtime a positive, nourishing experience filled with care and understanding.

Easing Sundowning Symptoms

Sundowning can be one of the more challenging and distressing parts of Alzheimer's care. As the afternoon turns into evening, you might notice that your loved one becomes more agitated, confused, or even aggressive. This change, known as sundowning, is common in the middle stages of Alzheimer's and can be hard for both of you.

Understanding that sundowning results from the worsening of dementia symptoms in the late afternoon and evening can help you better manage these changes. Factors like low lighting, increased shadows, and disruptions in the body's internal clock can contribute to this condition. Fading light can also increase confusion and fear.

To help reduce these symptoms, start by improving the lighting in your home as the day progresses. You don't need to make every room as bright as noon, but aim for a gentle increase in light to counteract the gloom of twilight. Use lamps with a soft glow to create a calming atmosphere. Reducing the contrast between light and dark areas can help lessen confusion and anxiety.

Reducing noise and clutter during this time can help decrease confusion and agitation. Turn off the TV or switch from distressing news channels to soothing music or nature shows. Keep the main living areas free of clutter and unnecessary distractions to create a peaceful environment that can help ease their mind.

Coming up with a calming evening routine can make a big difference in easing sundowning symptoms. This might include activities like listening to soft music, taking a warm bath, or engaging in a relaxing hobby such as knitting or doing puzzles. The key is consistency and calmness; a predictable routine can provide a sense of security and familiarity, reducing anxiety as night falls. Keep evening activities light and easy, avoiding complex tasks or discussions that could increase frustration and confusion.

Mary was quite social and loved having family and friends visit. Unfortunately, she started becoming very agitated around 5pm. Ken continued to invite people to visit because it gave Mary so much joy. He explained to the visitors that they

needed to leave at 4pm so that Mary would not become over-
whelmed. Ken came up with an evening routine using
aromatherapy and soft lighting to create a calm, peaceful home
environment. On days with no visitors, he would put nature
shows on TV with the sound off. Mary's sundowning symptoms
noticeably vanished as she got used to the routine.

Keeping a consistent sleep schedule and active daytime routine is also important. Exposure to natural light during the day can help regulate their internal clock, which is often disrupted in people with Alzheimer's. Include activities that encourage movement and engagement, whether it's a walk in the park or simple indoor exercises. These not only help reduce restlessness towards the evening but also promote better sleep quality. As night approaches, help your loved one wind down with a consistent bedtime routine. This could involve brushing teeth, changing into nightwear, and reading a story, playing soothing music, or engaging in prayer to signal it's time to sleep.

Implementing these strategies takes patience and observation. You might need to adjust routines as you figure out what best soothes and comforts your loved one during these twilight hours. Remember, each person with Alzheimer's is unique, and their response to different approaches can vary. It's about finding the right balance that offers them comfort and stability, reducing the impact of sundowning on their well-being.

Aggression Addressed Compassionately

Dealing with aggression in middle stage Alzheimer's can be one of the most challenging aspects of caregiving. Aggression may arise unexpectedly, triggered by factors such as physical discomfort, emotional distress, or changes in the environment. Recognizing these triggers is crucial as it allows you to address the root causes rather than just the symptoms. For example, pain from a medical condition like arthritis might manifest as aggression if it goes unexpressed. Similarly, emotional distress caused by too much noise, or a disrupted routine can lead to aggressive behaviors. Environmental factors, such as a cluttered room or poor lighting, can also contribute to confusion and aggression. Social engagements with large groups or noisy environments might cause agitation, so smaller, quieter gatherings might be more suitable. Telling them that they are wrong or forgot something, can raise their fear or anxiety and cause anger and aggression.

Keeping a detailed log of incidents can help you identify specific triggers by revealing patterns over time. This proactive approach allows you to modify routines or the environment to mitigate these triggers. For instance, ensuring the living space is calm, well-lit, and free from unnecessary clutter can create a more reassuring atmosphere, potentially reducing episodes of aggression.

Sophia never liked other people's belongings in her home and would regularly toss them aside when she found them. As her Alzheimer's symptoms progressed, she stopped recognizing her own clothing in the several closets she had. Sophia became convinced that someone was putting strangers' clothes in her closets. This led her to rip, cut up, and throw her clothes in the trash. Their daughter acknowledged Sophia's feelings and managed to convince her to donate the clothes instead of destroying them. This calmed Sophia down, and she agreed to work with her daughter to significantly reduce her closet until she was satisfied it was no longer cluttered, and she wanted to keep the remaining clothes.

De-escalation techniques can help you manage aggressive behaviors safely and effectively. The key is to remain calm. Remember, your loved one is likely reacting out of confusion or fear, so responding with distress can escalate the situation. Here are a few techniques to help manage aggression:

- **Stay Calm:** Speak in a soft, soothing tone, keeping your body language open and non-threatening.
- **Active Listening:** Pay attention to both verbal and non-verbal clues to understand what is causing the aggressive behavior.
- **Empathetic Communication:** Use empathetic statements to validate your loved one's feelings, even if you don't agree with their reasoning. Saying things like, "I can tell this is really upsetting you, why don't we take a break" acknowledges their feelings and can help de-escalate the situation by making them feel heard and understood. Avoid arguing or trying to reason with them during moments of aggression, as this can increase agitation.
- **Address the Need:** If possible, address the immediate cause of distress. This could involve turning on a light, moving an object, or resolving a complex task.
- **Distract and Redirect Them:** If aggression occurs during a specific activity, gently guide them to a different setting or engage them in a simpler activity to shift their focus and reduce stress.
- **Offer Reassuring Touch:** Physical touch, like a gentle hand on the shoulder, can sometimes reassure and calm down your loved one. However, be mindful of their response to touch, as they may be more sensitive about their personal space during aggressive episodes. Do not approach if they are physically lashing out. Keep yourself safe.
- **Put Safety First:** Make sure the environment is free of potential hazards. Maintain a safe distance to react quickly, but stay close enough to communicate and provide

reassurance. If their aggression escalates beyond your control, seek professional help. Have a plan in place for who to call, whether a family member, healthcare provider, or emergency services, to get timely assistance. This keeps both you and your loved one safe.

By using these compassionate techniques, you can better manage aggressive behaviors and create a safer, more supportive environment for your loved one.

Managing Delusions, Paranoia, and Hallucinations

In the midst of middle stage Alzheimer's, you might find yourself facing some of the most bewildering behaviors: delusions, paranoia, and hallucinations. These symptoms are distressing not only for your loved one but also for you as a caregiver. They stem from profound changes in the brain that affect perception and memory. As Alzheimer's progresses, it can warp the brain's ability to interpret sensory information correctly, leading to false perceptions or exaggerated beliefs. Environmental triggers like poor lighting or unfamiliar settings can make these issues worse, as can certain health problems or medication side effects. Understanding these root causes is the first step in managing these complex behaviors effectively.

Hallucinations involve sensory experiences that seem real but are not, such as hearing voices or seeing people who aren't there. Delusions in Alzheimer's might manifest as firmly held false beliefs that don't match reality, such as thinking family members are impostors. Paranoia, often accompanying delusions, may cause someone with Alzheimer's to believe they are being persecuted or harmed. Distinguishing between these symptoms is essential because it shapes how you respond. For example, reassuring someone experiencing paranoia might differ from redirecting someone distressed by hallucinations.

When responding to hallucinations, empathy is key. Recognize the reality of their experience without reinforcing the hallucination. For instance, if they mention seeing children playing in the living room when there are none, rather than bluntly denying the vision, acknowledge their experience and gently guide their attention elsewhere. You might suggest a walk outside or start a different activity like looking through a photo album. Maintaining a calm, soothing presence helps provide reassurance and can prevent the situation from escalating.

> *Jamal and Kalia's father, Winston, started having frequent episodes of believing strangers were trying to break into their home, as the evening hours approached. Jamal noticed the house became noticeably darker and evening winds and outside noises were easier to hear. Kalia put up black out curtains, which reduced the outside notices, and installed more blue and yellow lights throughout the house, so that it was evenly lit in more warm and calming colors. Jamal put the lights and Winston's favorite music on timers so the house never got too dark, and Winston had a distraction he enjoyed. When Winston thought he heard someone breaking in, one of his kids would start humming the song that was playing and Winston would join in. Winston felt safe and everyone felt less stress.*

Managing delusions and paranoia in someone with Alzheimer's requires creating a safe, secure environment that reduces anxiety and fear. Avoid arguing about their misconceptions, as this only increases agitation. Instead, focus on their feelings rather than the facts. If they claim someone has stolen something, acknowledge their distress and assure them of their safety. Then, gently redirect their attention to a different activity or topic. This approach helps manage immediate behavior while preserving their dignity and reducing anxiety.

Michele was certain that someone was stealing her valuables and hiding them. She would often blame her husband, because he would often find her valuables and return them to her. Michele decided that her husband was hiding her things to make her upset and torture her. Her grandson, Keiko would help her look for her items, and no matter where they were found, she would still blame her husband. Keiko asked his grandfather to install cameras around the house and garage where her items were normally lost. Now, when something is lost, Keiko and his grandfather will review the camera videos to discover where Michele hid her belongings. Then they would have Michele join them in the search of that room. This did not stop Michele from hiding her belongings, or blaming her husband, but it did stop the screaming, yelling, and aggression she would show when she felt persecuted. Now, when Michele loses something, she will call Keiko. He will review the videos on his phone and suggest places for her to search based on where he believes she hid her belongings. Keiko's grandfather is grateful that Michele is no longer angry and aggressive towards him when she loses something.

Knowing when to seek professional help is crucial. Monitor the frequency and intensity of these symptoms and how they impact your loved one's behavior and quality of life. If delusions, paranoia, or hallucinations become severe, consult healthcare professionals. They may need to adjust current medications or consider new ones to help manage symptoms more effectively. Professional guidance can provide additional strategies and support, ensuring you're not navigating these complex behaviors alone.

Communicating in the Middle Stage

As Alzheimer's progresses, it changes the way your loved one understands and uses language. Recognizing these changes is like noticing the subtle shifts in the seasons—it's not just the big changes, but the small ones too. Early signs that language is becoming more difficult might include losing track of conversations often, struggling to find the right word, or using simpler phrases and sentences. These changes mean it's time to adjust how you communicate to meet their evolving needs.

> *One day Elaine asked her husband for a glass of water. Robert asked if she wanted sparkling or still. Elaine didn't understand and asked what the difference was. Robert was perplexed and didn't answer at first. He didn't understand why she was asking. This question was part of their daily routine. He asked again, and Elaine asked which one was better. Robert realized this was one of the communication changes he needed to watch out for. He explained that sparkling water had little bubbles in it and the other water did not. Elaine said she liked bubbles and Robert smiled and got her a glass of sparkling water. Robert's realization after his initial surprise allowed Elaine to feel cared for, and stopped Robert from feeling frustrated.*

During this time, simplicity is your friend. As cognitive abilities decline, complex sentences and abstract ideas can become hard to understand. Simplifying your language doesn't mean talking down to your loved one; it means making communication easier. Break instructions into clear, manageable steps. For example, instead of saying, "Get ready for your appointment," you might say, "Time to put on your shoes," followed by, "Now, how about we grab your coat." This step-by-step approach makes it easier for them to follow along, reducing frustration and confusion.

As Alzheimer's advances, focusing on non-verbal cues becomes even more important. your loved one may rely more on facial expressions, body language, and other physical movements to show their feelings and needs. A furrowed brow might indicate confusion or worry, while a relaxed posture may show contentment. Paying attention to these signals can help you respond better to their emotional and physical needs. It's about creating a conversation without words that respects their current abilities and shows your constant support and understanding.

When your loved one shows signs of distress, like grimacing or withdrawing, respond with gentleness and reassurance. Calmness and empathy can go a long way. Sometimes, simply hearing comforting words in a soothing tone can help restore their peace. A gentle touch or a hand on the shoulder can communicate safety and compassion more effectively than words. These responses not only relieve immediate distress but also strengthens the emotional bond you share, reinforcing their sense of security and trust in your care.

Encouraging positive non-verbal interactions is also essential to emotional health. Simple actions like smiling, making eye contact, or sharing a gentle touch are universal ways to show care. They convey affection, reassurance, and presence, creating a positive emotional environment. Regularly engaging in these heartfelt interactions can improve their well-being, making them feel valued and connected despite the challenges of Alzheimer's.

Training and practice in these communication techniques can improve your effectiveness as a caregiver. Consider joining workshops or online courses focused on communication skills in dementia care. These training opportunities provide practical techniques and insights that can enrich your interactions with your loved one, making each conversation more meaningful and every response more attuned to their unique needs.

In the delicate dance of communication with your loved one, every gesture, word, and silence matters. By adapting your communication strategies and continually responding to their feedback, you can create a nurturing environment that respects their changing abilities and affirms their dignity. It's about speaking the language of Alzheimer's with compassion and clarity, ensuring that your loved one feels heard, understood, and deeply cared for throughout their journey.

Supportive Technology

Today, technology serves as a powerful tool in connecting with and caring for a person with Alzheimer's. These tools aren't just convenient—they can make a real difference in bridging gaps in communication.

Take large-button phones, for example. These phones have big, easy-to-read buttons and simple interfaces, making them perfect for someone who struggles with tiny, complex gadgets. The feel of actual buttons can be comforting for those who find touchscreens overwhelming. Similarly, photo dial phones let you set contacts with pictures, so your loved one can easily call family and friends by pressing a photo. This can help them feel more independent and connected.

Voice-activated devices, like smart speakers, and cell phones can also be very helpful. These devices respond to simple voice commands, letting your loved one make phone calls, set reminders, or play music without dealing with complicated buttons and menus. Introducing these devices requires patience and a gradual approach. Start by showing basic functions and encourage your loved one to try simple commands, praising their efforts to build confidence.

Dorena felt a need to keep her possessions safe, so her brother,

Mike got her a biometric safe. This way, she didn't have to worry about lost keys or forgetting the combination. All she had to do was place her finger over the scanner to open the safe. As Dorena's cognitive skills declined, she still remembered how to open and lock the safe for quite some time, as it was a skill embedded in her body like opening a door or turning on a faucet. Eventually, Dorena started leaving the safe open and wondering who else had a "key" to her safe, but for some time, it reduced the hiding of important items like her wallet and medications.

There are also many apps designed specifically for dementia care. These apps often use visual aids and easy interfaces to improve understanding and engagement. Some apps have memory games that keep the brain active and are fun to play. Others help improve communication by using pictures and simple phrases to help users express their needs and feelings. Apps like 'TalkingMats' use pictures and symbols to help individuals express their needs, feelings, and preferences. This visual method can be very effective, tapping into the brain's ability to recognize and process images even as verbal abilities decline. When choosing these tools, pick ones that match your loved one's current abilities and interests so that they are both useful and enjoyable.

Speech-generating devices allow users to input their thoughts and feelings, which are then spoken aloud by the device.

Video calls have changed how we stay connected, especially when visits aren't possible. Seeing a familiar face on the screen can provide much-needed emotional comfort for your loved one. When setting up video calls, make sure the environment is quiet and the setup is simple. Try to keep calls at a regular time to maintain a routine. During the call, talk about familiar topics and give your loved one plenty of time to respond, even if it's just with smiles or gestures.

These interactions can bring joy and remind them of the love and connections that remain strong despite the challenges.

The key to using technology effectively is to customize it to fit the needs of your loved one. This might mean setting up devices with larger text, adjusting screen brightness, or changing audio settings for better hearing. Choose technology that aligns with what they are used to and comfortable with. If your loved one has always used a certain type of phone or computer, finding similar devices can reduce frustration and make the transition smoother.

Incorporating technology into Alzheimer's care is about more than just gadgets and apps. It's about improving quality of life, maintaining dignity, and opening up new ways to communicate and interact. These tools can become essential parts of the caregiving experience, enriching the lives of both you and your loved one.

Late Stage Alzheimer's Care

L ate stage Alzheimer's is a tender chapter in which the essence of caregiving shifts significantly. It's no longer about managing a schedule or making sure medications are taken on time. Now, it's about creating a sanctuary of comfort and filling each moment with as much peace and familiarity as possible. Maintaining your loved one's dignity and comfort becomes your primary concern. Here, in the soft twilight of their cognitive abilities, your role transcends basic care—it becomes a profound act of love and respect.

The Evolution of Late Stage Alzheimer's

In stages 6 and 7 of Alzheimer's, the complexities of care evolve dramatically. Your loved one may no longer communicate with words, and their world—as they perceive it—might seem vastly different from your own. Yet, they continue to experience emotions; they feel joy, discomfort, fear, and love, even if their expressions of these feelings have changed. They might no longer speak clearly or recognize familiar faces, but they respond to the tone of your voice, the touch of your hand, and the comfort of your presence.

Creating an emotionally safe space becomes your top priority. This involves more than physical safety—it's about nurturing a space where they can feel secure and loved. Visual and tactile stimulation plays a critical role in this. Simple gestures like keeping family photos nearby, arranging their room with favorite objects, or letting them hold a well-loved item can spark moments of joy or recognition. Engaging their senses with soft, familiar music, the scent of a favorite meal, or the texture of a cherished blanket can provide comfort even when words fail.

Emotional engagement is imperative, even if it feels like your efforts are not being acknowledged. Talking to your loved one, sharing stories from the past, or simply sitting with them in silence can all provide comfort and a sense of normalcy. Social interactions should be maintained, although adjusted to their current capabilities. Small, quiet gatherings with close family or friends can be soothing, provided they don't cause overstimulation. It's important to read their cues—if they seem restless or upset, it might be best to limit interactions to one-on-one or smaller, quieter settings.

Remember, someone with Alzheimer's can still perceive more than we might realize. They may catch on to stress or sadness in your voice or become peaceful from the calmness in your touch. Their ability to process complex sentences or follow logical narratives may seem to have disappeared, but their fundamental human instincts for emotional connection remain. Your presence, filled with patience and empathy, reassures them that they are not alone, providing a profound sense of security and belonging.

Navigating late stage Alzheimer's requires a deep well of compassion and resilience. It's about finding balance—knowing when to hold on to the routines that provide comfort, and when to let go, allowing moments to unfold naturally, guided by the needs and responses of your loved one. In this stage, every small act of care is a reaffirmation of their dignity and proof of your enduring love for them. As you adapt your strategies and prepare to meet their changing needs, remember that this phase, while challenging, can also be a deeply meaningful time of connection that honors the fullness of their life's journey.

Changes to Daily Living

As the disease progresses into the late stages, you may find yourself needing to assist more and more with the daily care needs, until you find yourself completely responsible for all of them. The caregiving needs are made more difficult by your loved one's increasing decline in motor skills and ability to walk, stand, or transfer to a wheelchair. Physical difficulties like trouble chewing or swallowing can make eating exhausting and uncomfortable. There may be a marked decrease in movement and agitation, but the daily activities of living have become more intense.

You may experience some of the following progressions:

- Helping your loved one use to the bathroom, to changing diapers in a bed
- From handing them their toothbrush to brushing their teeth
- From having them participate in their grooming, to you doing it all
- Helping your loved one get dressed, to dressing your loved one
- Helping your loved one bathe, to bathing your loved one, to sponge baths in bed
- From cutting up food, to having lots of finger food, to feeding your loved one
- From offering regular food, to soft food, to pureed food

- Helping them eat 3 regular meals per day which increases in time from 30 - 90 minutes each meal, to offering food every couple of hours for about 30 minutes per session
- From watching them walk, to providing support like a walker, to helping them walk, to using a wheelchair to eventually leaving them in bed because they can no longer sit up in a wheelchair
- With the wheelchair you may progress from directing them to stand and swivel, to helping them stand and swivel, to using a Hoyer lift (a machine that lifts them up and places them, for example, in the wheelchair or bed)
- From listening to them be challenged finding words, to listening to gibberish, to discovering they are no longer speaking

If your loved one is still living at home, this is the time when you most need to have at least one additional regular caregiver. This may mean partnering with other family members, friends, or even hiring private caregivers.

Pain Management

In the late stages of Alzheimer's, your role as a caregiver becomes less about conversation and active engagement and more about creating a serene environment that soothes and comforts.

Pain management, a core aspect of late stage care, often presents a challenge since your loved one may no longer communicate discomfort in ways that are easy to understand. Recognizing non-verbal cues of pain—such as grimacing, restlessness, or a sudden withdrawal from usual activities—is vital. These subtle signs can indicate discomfort that, if unaddressed, might lead to severe distress.

Physical comfort can be managed through regular assessments for pain or discomfort, gentle daily exercise to prevent muscle stiffness, and ensuring they are always comfortably seated or lying down. Use pillows for support, keep their living space at a comfortable temperature, and be vigilant about potential sources of pain or discomfort, like tight clothing or skin irritations.

Regular consultations with healthcare professionals allow for adjustments in pain management protocols, helping to keep your loved one comfortable without overusing medications that could cause additional confusion or sedation.

Creating a soothing environment is equally crucial and involves more than just physical adjustments. It's about crafting a space that feels safe and familiar. Use soft, ambient lighting to create a calm atmosphere and minimize shadows or harsh lights that might cause confusion or fear. Keep the room at a comfortable temperature, considering that older adults often feel colder. Introduce familiar objects that can bring comfort and trigger positive memories, such as a favorite blanket, a well-loved book, or family photographs placed where they can see them easily. These familiar items can provide a sense of security and continuity, which is vital as their cognitive abilities decline.

The power of sensory stimulation in providing comfort cannot be overstated. Touch, in particular, is a profound way to communicate care and affection when words no longer suffice. Gentle hand massages, brushing their hair, or simply holding their hand can be incredibly comforting. Aromatherapy can also play a role in creating a calming environment; scents like lavender or chamomile can help alleviate anxiety and promote relaxation. Soft, melodic music can have a remarkably soothing effect, reducing stress and potentially improving cognitive function through the stimulation of rhythmic brain activity.

In managing late stage Alzheimer's, remember that your efforts in creating a comforting, respectful environment are invaluable. They not only enhance the quality of life for your loved one, but also help in managing the inevitable challenges that come with this stage of the disease. By focusing on pain management, environmental comfort, sensory stimulation, and dignified end-of-life care, you provide a level of care that goes beyond mere necessities, offering love, respect, and comfort during the most challenging times.

Staying Connected During Severe Memory Loss

As Alzheimer's progresses into its later stages, maintaining a connection with your loved one can seem increasingly challenging. They may no longer recognize you or respond to conversations as they once did, which can feel disheartening. However, remember that their need for love and connection remains unchanged.

> *Thom and Marcia loved to dance. Marcia had declined to the point where she could no longer stand or direct her arm movements, and she rarely showed any emotions. One day, the song they danced to at their wedding started to play. Thom locked eyes with Marcia, stood up, and pretended he was dancing with her. Marcia watched intently. A big smile slowly spread across her face as she watched Thom perform their wedding dance for her. It was the first time he'd seen her smile in over a week, and he smiled back at her with loving, tear-filled eyes.*

One profoundly effective method to reach through the fog of memory loss is reminiscence therapy. This technique involves evoking memories using tangible prompts from the past—photographs, favorite music, or cherished personal items. (This technique is detailed in the Compassionate Care section.) Engaging the senses can dramatically improve interactions for your loved one.

Incorporating elements that stimulate smell, touch, and sight can evoke responses even when verbal communication has faded.

Tactile activities like handling fabrics with different textures or engaging in gentle hand massage can provide comforting stimulation. Children's books, or books made for people with dementia, that have fabric swatches and other safe textures can keep your loved one occupied for quite some time. These sensory experiences offer them meaningful ways to connect with the world around them.

At this special time, your presence—calm, patient, and reassuring—becomes a foundation of comfort and familiarity amidst the confusion. Remember, it's not about recreating the past but about making each present moment as rich and comforting as possible. Through your efforts in managing pain, using reminiscence therapy, and engaging the senses, you provide not just care but a continued affirmation of their dignity and worth.

Advanced Communication Tips

As Alzheimer's progresses into its severe stages, you might find that the ways you used to communicate with your loved one aren't as effective as they once were. Words may no longer suffice, and their ability to express thoughts verbally might diminish significantly. In fact, they may start speaking what is gibberish to our ears, and finally, stop speaking altogether.

However, this doesn't lessen the importance of communication; it changes how it should be approached. Emphasizing non-verbal communication becomes imperative. Simple gestures like maintaining eye contact or offering a warm smile can help your loved one feel seen and understood, even if they're unable to express their thoughts verbally. Pointing to objects or showing actions, can reinforce your words, providing a multi-sensory way to communicate that's often easier to grasp.

Using touch—a gentle hand on the shoulder or holding their hand—can communicate comfort and reassurance more powerfully than words. Paying attention to your body language, ensuring it conveys openness and affection, helps maintain a strong emotional connection. These non-verbal cues often speak directly to the emotional center of the brain, which remains active even as other cognitive functions decline.

Creating a visually clear and simple environment can also significantly aid communication. Clutter and chaos can be confusing and distressing for someone with severe Alzheimer's. Simplifying their surroundings can help minimize confusion and make it easier for them to focus and find comfort in the familiarity of the space. This might mean keeping the living area tidy and organized, using simple decorations, and maintaining a consistent layout so that they can move through the space more intuitively. Labeling drawers and cabinets with pictures or simple words describing their contents can help your loved one find things they need independently, fostering a sense of control and self-reliance.

Navigating communication in the severe stages of Alzheimer's requires patience, creativity, and a willingness to adapt to new methods. Each adjustment you make can have a profound impact on your ability to stay connected, helping your loved one feel valued, understood, and cared for, even as communication becomes more challenging.

Symptom Management with Palliative Care

As caregiving shifts from handling new behaviors to focusing on comfort and quality of life, palliative care provides gentle, supportive care that truly prioritizes those needs. You may have heard the term "palliative care" and wondered what it really means. In essence, this type of care is all about easing the symptoms and stress of serious illnesses like Alzheimer's. It's not about curing the disease but about providing comfort and support, aiming to make your loved one's final years as peaceful and pain-free as possible.

The Palliative Care Team of doctors, nurses, social workers, and chaplains work alongside your other medical providers. Palliative Care doctors and nurses can greatly improve your loved one's quality of life by managing distressing symptoms such as pain, difficulty breathing, and agitation. Palliative Care Chaplains address the emotional, spiritual, or religious needs for both your loved one and the family. Palliative Care Social Workers may provide information about community resources like in-home podiatrists or hairdressers, private caregivers, caregiver support groups, and obtaining in-home medical equipment.

Managing symptoms in palliative care requires a compassionate mix of medical treatments and holistic therapies. Pain, a common issue in late stage Alzheimer's, can be tough to manage because your loved one might struggle to communicate their discomfort. A combination of prescribed medications and non-drug approaches like massage or music therapy can be effective. Massage helps relieve muscle stiffness and promote relaxation, while music therapy can calm agitation and improve emotional well-being. Aromatherapy with essential oils like lavender or chamomile can also help create a soothing environment, reduce anxiety, and improve sleep.

The heart of palliative care is its focus on the needs and wishes of your loved one and their family, ensuring that care is provided with dignity and respect. It's about making each day as good as it can be— physically, emotionally, and spiritually. As you navigate this delicate phase of care, remember that your efforts provide comfort and reassurance during a crucial time in your loved one's life. Each gentle touch, soothing word, and effort to ease discomfort shows your deep commitment to their dignity and well-being during their final journey.

Implementing an End-of-Life Care Plan

Creating an end-of-life care plan is a critical step in making sure your loved one's final wishes are respected and fulfilled. Ideally, you've already discussed these important decisions with your loved one and family during the early stages of the disease. Now that you understand your loved one's wishes and have documented them, it's time to reference those decisions and put an end-of-life plan into place.

When starting this conversation with family members, approach it with empathy and clarity, ensuring everyone feels supported. Choose a quiet, private time when you're not likely to be interrupted. Approach the conversation with gentleness, recognizing that while it's a difficult topic, it's important for respecting and fulfilling your loved one's wishes. Use clear, straightforward language and give the family time to express their feelings and thoughts. Everyone involved must understand that the goal of this discussion is not to hasten the farewell but to make the remaining time as meaningful and true to your loved one's wishes as possible.

Developing an end-of-life care plan includes making key decisions about the type of care desired in the final stages of life, such as when to transition from palliative care to hospice care, and what specific medical interventions, if any, should be avoided. This is also the time to remind family members of your loved one's decisions and ensure that these decisions are honored as much as possible.

Addressing emotional and spiritual considerations during this phase is imperative. Each family member will have their own needs and preferences when it comes to spiritual comfort. Focus on your loved one's preferences when addressing their care, rather than your own beliefs. Family members should also seek emotional and spiritual support from their own communities to help process the grief that may arise long before your loved one passes.

For many, this time might also stir profound questions about meaning, value, and connection. Chaplains are invaluable at this time to help facilitate discussions about your spirit, that is your emotional being and character, or faith based conversations, or helping you process grief. Pastoral counseling from your faith tradition is a great option to help you be in alignment with your specific religious beliefs. These services offer a space to process feelings and find peace, whether through structured therapy or more informal support and listening.

When to Transition to Hospice

Transitioning to hospice care can be a deeply emotional experience, and understanding when and how to make this transition is crucial. There are many misconceptions about hospice, so here are some useful facts to help clarify what hospice care involves:

- Hospice is typically recommended when a person is considered to be in the final six months of their life.
- Hospice can be provided in the home, in a facility, or wherever your loved one is living.
- Hospice provides in-home medical services, including doctors, nurses, social workers, hospice aides, and chaplains. They provide medical and emotional support when you and your loved one can no longer travel to a clinic.
- Hospice offers support by providing the necessary palliative care, medications, and in-home equipment like hospital

beds, walkers, and commodes to keep your loved one comfortable.

- Hospice focuses on comfort care rather than curative treatment.
- If your loved one has an infection, wound, or other issue causing discomfort, hospice can provide evaluation and treatment to maintain their comfort.
- Hospice does not cover care aimed at extending life, improving your loved one's condition, or diagnostic testing for diseases related to the six-month prognosis.
- If you want to try curative treatments, you will need to "revoke" hospice, which involves signing paperwork to discontinue hospice services.
- Hospice does not provide caregivers. Families must arrange for this support themselves.
- Hospice aides might visit one to three times a week for about 30-60 minutes to assist caregivers with personal care tasks like bathing or shaving. Hospice aides do not replace the caregiver's work of providing daily care needs. Their availability depends on the hospice organization's staffing and your family's needs.
- Hospice teams regularly evaluate patients, and if your loved one's condition improves, they may "graduate" from hospice care. This should never be a surprise, as your hospice team should keep you regularly informed. If you are concerned that your loved one might graduate, simply ask the nurse. Clear and direct communication is encouraged.

Discussing what hospice care involves can help demystify the process and alleviate some anxieties. It's also a time to reflect on what has been meaningful about your loved one's life, celebrating those memories, and reinforcing the love and connections that persist.

Managing this phase of care demands deep compassion and courage. It involves providing comfort, honoring wishes, and upholding dignity at every step. As you engage in these delicate conversations, develop care plans, and provide emotional and spiritual support, remember that each step taken is deeply valued. It's a profound service to your loved one, ensuring their preferences are respected and their legacy honored in the most loving way possible. As you continue to provide care, let these principles guide you, creating a space where peace, dignity, and love are the foundations of every interaction.

Transitioning Care Settings

When the care needs of your loved one evolve, transitioning between different care settings or levels of care can sometimes become necessary. Planning these transitions thoughtfully is crucial, not only for maintaining continuity and quality of care but also for preserving your loved one's dignity and comfort. Whether the transition is from home to a care facility or between different care levels within a facility, each move can be disorienting for your loved one. Therefore, involving them in decisions about their care, as much as they are able to participate, becomes a key aspect of preserving their autonomy and dignity.

> *Luis faced a tough situation when his older brother, Edgar, needed to move to a specialized care facility. In their close-knit family, taking care of each other was a deeply held value. So, while this decision brought relief, it was accompanied by a mountain of guilt. One afternoon, a nurse from the facility called to discuss the transition. Sensing Luis's worry, she shared a story about another family who found peace there, reassuring Luis that he was ensuring the best care for Edgar, not abandoning him. The nurse shared with him how Edgar's new*

room could be personalized with his favorite photos, movies, and books. She reminded him that frequent visits would keep their family bond strong. This compassionate approach made the move smoother for both brothers, helping Edgar feel at home and easing Luis's guilt.

Plan transitions carefully and in advance whenever possible to avoid unexpected stress. Discuss the potential need for future transitions early on, so it doesn't come as a surprise. Prepare a checklist of what will be needed for the transition, including personal items that will make the new environment feel familiar and comforting. If a move to a facility is necessary, try to involve your loved one in the selection process. Show them pictures of the facility, or if possible, take them for a visit. Seeing the new environment can help ease anxiety about the move and make the transition smoother.

Maintaining dignity in new care settings is about respecting and preserving the routines, preferences, and privacy of your loved one. When transitioning to a facility, make sure the staff is informed about their likes, dislikes, and any specific needs or routines that contribute to their comfort and sense of self. For example, if they prefer to have meals at a certain time or enjoy certain activities, communicate this to the caregivers. Additionally, personal care activities should be conducted with respect for their privacy and dignity. Simple actions like knocking before entering their room, addressing them by their preferred name, and involving them in daily care decisions as much as possible can make a significant difference in how they perceive their new living situation.

Building positive relationships with new caregivers or staff is essential for ensuring that your loved one receives compassionate and person-alized care. Initiate open communication with caregivers from the start. Share detailed information about your loved one's history, their likes and dislikes, and any nuances in their care needs. Regularly spending time at the facility and participating in care activities can help you build rapport with the staff and also keep you informed about the care your loved one is receiving. Encourage staff to share observations about your loved one's condition and behavior, as this can provide insights that might help in adjusting care plans.

Regular visits and interactions are not just about monitoring the quality of care; they also play a critical role in helping your loved one adjust to the new environment. During visits, engage in activities that your loved one enjoys, bring familiar items from home, and spend quality time interacting with them. This continuity of family presence reminds them of the love and support they have, which can be incredibly reassuring in a new setting. Don't forget to be proactive in advocating for your loved one. If you notice anything that might improve their comfort or well-being, discuss it with the care team. Being actively involved in this way helps ensure that the care setting not only meets their medical needs but also enriches their life and respects their dignity.

Transitioning care settings is a significant step that can be approached with sensitivity and careful planning. By involving your loved one in decisions, maintaining their dignity, building strong relationships with caregivers, and staying actively involved in their care, you create a supportive environment that respects their needs and preferences. This thoughtful approach not only smooths the transition but also helps your loved one continue to feel valued and cared for, regardless of where they are in their Alzheimer's journey.

Section Three
Compassionate Care

Imagine walking into a room that you're certain you've never been in before, but something about it feels familiar, comforting, and pleasurable. This is the challenge your loved one faces as the memories fade, but the emotional experiences remain.

> *David was in the late stages of Alzheimer's and rarely spoke anymore. His whole life once revolved around music and the choirs he sang in. One day, his husband, Jim, was flipping through an album of pictures with David, and they found an anniversary picture. Feeling nostalgic, Jim played the song David used to sing to him every year on that special day. Out of nowhere, David started singing along—getting every word right— and smiled at Jim as he finished the song. Just as quickly, David's face went back to its neutral expression, but that was a moment Jim never forgot.*

These are the experiences you want to invite your loved one to have as often as possible, and the moments compassionate care aims to bring about. Compassionate care is more than just meeting physical needs—it's about nurturing the whole person, respecting their life story, and finding ways to rekindle the things that still bring them joy.

Caring For the Whole Person

Compassionate care means paying close attention to every aspect of a person's life, including their social, cultural, familial, and spiritual well-being. It's about seeing the person behind the condition and tailoring your care to fit their entire being. This holistic approach not only improves the quality of care but also enriches the lives of both the caregiver and the loved one they've taken under their wing.

Compassionate care is built on a foundation of empowerment for your loved one. It involves recognizing and nurturing their abilities, whatever they may be, to foster autonomy and self-worth. For instance, if the person was once an avid gardener, encouraging them to engage in simple gardening tasks can fill them with purpose and joy. Maybe they can't manage the heavy tools anymore, but they can still help with planting seeds or deadheading flowers. These activities are not just tasks; they're connections to their past and anchors to their present.

In the home, minor modifications like automatic night lights that illuminate paths to the bathroom or lever-style door handles can make a tremendous difference in their ability to confidently move through the space.

Finding the balance between safety and independence is one of the trickiest parts of Alzheimer's care. It's natural to want to protect your loved one from harm, but overly restrictive measures can diminish their independence and dignity. The goal is to find that sweet spot where they are safe but not confined. For example, instead of restricting all kitchen activities, you might introduce safe appliances that allow them to prepare basic meals without posing a risk. This idea can be applied to almost any other hobby of theirs, which may still be an integral part of their identity, even in this season of life.

> *Annaleise used to own a wedding cake business and was a proud baker, but her declining motor skills made it tough for her to use utensils and appliances. Wanting to support Annaleise's passion, her daughter Rebecca made some changes to the kitchen. Rebecca brought in easy-grip cooking tools. She instituted "Friday bake days" and would set up a baking station with things in easy reach of Annaleise. Annaleise loved spending Fridays sharing her passion with her daughter. Baking in partnership allowed Rebecca to do the tasks her mother no longer could, and brought them both joy and a sense of normalcy.*

Focusing on these aspects of compassionate care can help you create a nurturing environment that respects and honors your loved one as a whole person. As their abilities shift, you will need to shift your approach to how you incorporate these approaches in their life. Compassionate care heightens their quality of life and ensures your loved one feels valued and understood. In turn, you gain a deeper appreciation for the person they are, which can turn your experience as a caregiver from one of duty to one of meaningful connection and mutual respect.

Understanding Cultural Differences

Professional caregivers need to understand how different cultural backgrounds shape the caregiving experience. Family caregivers should work with professional caregivers to help them understand the cultural influences relevant to your loved one. Cultural beliefs about health, illness, and caregiving deeply influence how families respond to an Alzheimer's diagnosis and the care that follows.

In some cultures, diseases like Alzheimer's are seen not just as medical issues but also as spiritual or familial challenges that the whole family is expected to handle. This can affect how symptoms are viewed and treated, influencing everything from accepting the diagnosis to following medical advice. Some communities might prefer traditional health practices over modern medicine or emphasize natural remedies and holistic health approaches, which should be respectfully included in the care plan if desired.

Mrs. Kim's twins, Maya and Cho, found that combining traditional Korean medicine with modern treatments made a significant difference in their mother's life. Mrs. Kim believed strongly in the healing power of herbal remedies and acupuncture, which she had used all her life. Maya and Cho were determined to honor their mother's beliefs and traditions. They worked with her healthcare team to incorporate these practices into her care plan, creating a treatment that was a blend of both worlds. This approach not only made Mrs. Kim feel respected and comfortable but also brought a sense of familiarity and peace to her daily routine.

Cultural norms also determine who becomes the caregiver and what their duties include. In many cultures, caregiving is seen as a family responsibility, often falling on women or the eldest child. This can put a lot of emotional and physical stress on the caregiver, especially if they don't have enough support from other family members or their community. Understanding these dynamics is a fundamental part of providing culturally sensitive care and supporting the caregivers themselves. Discussing these cultural expectations openly can help families share caregiving duties more fairly, reducing stress and preventing burnout.

Attitudes toward aging and end-of-life care are also shaped by cultural beliefs. Some cultures have deep respect for the elderly, viewing age as a sign of wisdom and making caring for older family members a duty of honor. This can influence decisions about end-of-life care, with a strong preference for keeping elderly relatives at home rather than in care facilities. On the other hand, some cultures might trust professional care facilities more for providing the specialized care needed in the later stages of Alzheimer's. Respectfully addressing these different perspectives ensures that care decisions honor cultural values and family wishes.

Communication is another area where cultural nuances play a significant role. Language barriers can make the already challenging task of caregiving even more difficult. Even when families speak the same language as healthcare providers, cultural differences in communication styles can lead to misunderstandings. Using culturally and linguistically appropriate services is crucial. This might involve using interpreters or translators during medical appointments or having healthcare professionals trained in cultural competence to keep all communications clear and effective. This approach helps build trust and understanding between families and medical teams, making the caregiving journey smoother and more effective.

Navigating the cultural aspects of compassionate care requires sensitivity, understanding, and a willingness to learn and adapt. By accepting and integrating the cultural values and beliefs of your loved one and the family, caregivers can provide care that is not only effective but also respectful and affirming. It is vital that you share this information with professional caregivers and the medical team. This cultural awareness enriches the caregiving experience, creating a deeper connection and mutual respect between caregivers, family members, and your loved one.

Personalizing Care by Background

This chapter is for professional caregivers. If you are not a professional caregiver, but planning on hiring a private caregiver or working with a facility. Please share this chapter with them.

Caring for someone with Alzheimer's means understanding more than just their medical needs. This is especially important when you think about the different cultural backgrounds families come from. For professional caregivers, starting with a cultural assessment is like mapping out a journey in unfamiliar terrain. It involves understanding the person with Alzheimer's and their family's language preferences, religious beliefs, dietary restrictions, and other cultural details that might affect their care. This first step is key because it helps create a care plan that respects and honors the cultural identity of the one you will be caring for.

Imagine preparing a meal for guests from different cultures. You'd want to choose dishes that reflect their culinary preferences and dietary restrictions, right? Similarly, when you incorporate cultural preferences into daily care routines for someone with Alzheimer's, you make their care feel as comforting as a favorite family recipe. This could mean preparing meals that fit their traditional dietary practices or including specific rituals that they find spiritually fulfilling. For instance, if a person with Alzheimer's finds peace in prayer or medita-tion, making sure they have a quiet space for these practices can significantly improve their daily routine.

Training in cultural competence can help you provide respectful and understanding care. Whether you are a professional or family care-giver, understanding the subtle differences in cultures can greatly improve the care you give. It's more than just avoiding misunder-standings—it's about building trust and empathy. Engaging in training programs focused on cultural sensitivity can give you the knowledge and skills needed to navigate this complex part of care. Also, using resources like support groups and community organiza-tions that serve specific cultural groups can provide practical support and valuable insights into the best care practices for people from diverse backgrounds.

Creating an inclusive environment in professional care settings ensures that everyone feels understood and valued, no matter their cultural background. This can be achieved in several ways. Cele-brating a variety of cultural holidays can make the care environment more welcoming. Displaying decorations or artwork that reflects different cultures can help people with Alzheimer's feel more at home. Hiring staff from diverse cultural backgrounds or who speak multiple languages can also greatly improve the care experience. This diversity not only makes people feel respected but also enriches the care environment, making it a place where multiple perspectives are celebrated and where everyone can learn from each other.

By weaving cultural sensitivity and awareness into Alzheimer's care, you provide more than just physical care—you care for the person's soul. Acknowledging and respecting their life story, heritage, and identity can greatly enrich their experience and give them the comfort and dignity they deserve.

Staying Socially Connected

Picture the soothing melody of a familiar song, light conversation, and laughter filling the room. These aren't merely pleasant sounds; rather, they fulfill fundamental needs for someone with Alzheimer's. Social interactions are essential for their well-being, helping to lift their mood, stimulate their mind, and provide a sense of normalcy and belonging. On the other hand, isolation can worsen Alzheimer's symptoms, increasing confusion, anxiety, and speeding up cognitive decline. Social interactions offer a break from these challenges, helping them feel connected and remembered.

Adapting social activities for your loved one requires thought and creativity. It's about making sure these gatherings are safe, enjoyable, and inclusive. Hosting smaller quieter gatherings can be less overwhelming than large, noisy parties. In these settings, a person with Alzheimer's can interact more meaningfully with others, making it less confusing and more manageable. Structured activities like music therapy sessions, gentle group exercise classes, or simple craft projects can provide both social and mental stimulation. These activities should match their abilities. For example, a sing-along with old favorites can bring back memories and encourage participation, while a group exercise class designed for older adults can help maintain their physical health without being too difficult.

Using community resources can also help keep your loved one engaged. Many communities have senior centers or Alzheimer's associations that offer programs specifically for people with dementia, including art classes and gentle physical activities. Religious groups or clubs can also provide a sense of community and routine, which is comforting for someone with Alzheimer's. Joining these programs not only enriches their daily life but also gives you, as a caregiver, a much-needed break, helping you avoid burnout.

Encouraging visits from family and friends is crucial for maintaining social connections. However, make sure visitors know how to interact with your loved one. Simple strategies can make these visits more enjoyable and less stressful for everyone involved. For instance, reminding visitors to approach your loved one calmly, speak clearly, and bring up familiar topics can make a big difference. Encouraging visitors to bring items that might interest your loved one, like photos or a favorite album, can help spark conversation. Preparing visitors for any potential changes in behavior or memory can help manage expectations, making the visit more pleasant for both your guests and your loved one.

By thoughtfully planning interactions, adapting activities, using community resources, and educating family and friends, you can provide a richer, more joyful life for your loved one. These social engagements are vital in their care, offering moments of connection that are as helpful as any medicine.

Therapeutic Activities for All Stages

When caring for someone with advanced Alzheimer's, it's easy to focus on practical tasks like managing medications, ensuring safety, and keeping a routine. However, engaging all of their senses is just as important at every stage. Sensory activities can bring emotional comfort and create moments of connection that go beyond memory loss. These activities use the five senses to create positive feelings, calm agitation, and provide comfort. For someone who might not be able to communicate well, sensory experiences can be a way to connect and bring joy.

Take aromatherapy, for example. Scents can have a powerful effect on the brain, especially those tied to emotions and memories. Using familiar and pleasant scents like lavender, which is calming, or peppermint, which is refreshing, can quickly improve mood and well-being. You can set up a diffuser with these essential oils in the living room or use scented lotions during personal care routines. This can turn everyday activities into sensory experiences that comfort and sometimes even bring back memories. Just be careful to use these scents sparingly and make sure they're not too strong, always considering any allergies or sensitivities.

Tactile activities are another great way to engage someone with Alzheimer's. For someone who loves gardening, a tray filled with soil and small plants can provide a soothing touch of nature and keep their hands busy. Fabric swatches with different textures—like silk, corduroy, or velvet—can be interesting to touch and manipulate. Even simple water play, such as washing plastic cups, can be calming and engaging. These activities not only stimulate the sense of touch but also help maintain fine motor skills and hand-eye coordination.

Tailoring activities to your loved one's history and interests makes these moments even more special. For example, consider a husband and wife who loved to ballroom dance. In the early stages of Alzheimer's, they might still enjoy dancing together to their favorite music, even if it's just simple steps in the living room. As the disease progresses, they can adapt by dancing while seated or simply holding hands and gently swaying. Eventually, watching old tapes may be the only way to revisit those moments. For your loved one, seeing those cherished memories on video can bring a rare smile to their face, sparking joy for both of them and connecting them to you and their past.

Through these therapeutic activities and engagements, you're not just passing the time; you're enriching it. You're acknowledging that despite the cognitive decline, the heart and the senses can still enjoy, connect, and find comfort in the world around them. This approach doesn't just care for your loved one; it honors them, celebrating their life and legacy in every activity, touch, and scent.

Cognitive Games and Brain Activities

Engaging someone with Alzheimer's in cognitive exercises isn't just about passing time; it also helps keep their brain healthy and can slow cognitive decline. These activities, when matched to their abilities and interests, can bring joy and a sense of accomplishment while supporting their brain function. Think of these exercises as a workout for the brain, much like physical exercise benefits the body.

Choosing the right cognitive games and activities is key and should be based on your loved one's current cognitive abilities and past interests. For example, if they enjoyed puzzles, they might find satisfaction in jigsaw puzzles with larger, easier-to-handle pieces. For those who liked numbers, simple math games can be a stimulating challenge. Matching games, memory games, and basic board games not only offer fun but also help with pattern recognition and problem-solving skills. The games should be challenging enough to exercise the brain but not so hard that they cause frustration.

Apps like 'Lumosity' and 'CogniFit' offer games and activities designed to challenge and improve cognitive skills. Based on the principles of neuroplasticity, engaging in these activities can help maintain cognitive function for longer. These tools provide a variety of games targeting different cognitive skills such as memory, attention, and problem-solving, making cognitive stimulation a fun and rewarding part of the day.

Regular cognitive stimulation has well-documented benefits. Studies show that mentally stimulating activities can improve brain function and maintain neural connections. It's like keeping a car engine running smoothly by driving it regularly. For someone with Alzheimer's, regular mental exercises can help preserve existing cognitive functions and possibly slow the disease's progression. This regular stimulation can also provide a sense of normalcy and routine, which is comforting as they face the challenges of Alzheimer's.

Incorporating these activities into the daily routine should be done thoughtfully. Setting aside a specific time each day for these activities can help establish a routine and make it something the person looks forward to. This could be a morning session of card games or a post-lunch puzzle time. The key is consistency and making these activities a regular part of their day. Involving other family members or friends in these activities can increase enjoyment and effectiveness through social interaction.

As the disease progresses, the types and complexities of the activities will need to be adjusted. Simplifying games or switching to different activities that require less cognitive effort can help maintain engagement without causing frustration. For example, if complex puzzles become too difficult, switching to simpler sorting tasks or color matching can provide an alternative that still offers cognitive benefits. The focus should always be on the process and enjoyment rather than the outcome of these activities. Celebrating the effort and participation rather than success in these games can help maintain a positive experience and encourage continued engagement.

By carefully selecting and adapting cognitive activities, you provide not just mental stimulation but also a way to connect with your loved one, offering moments of joy and achievement that are invaluable in the journey of Alzheimer's care. Getting them involved in activities they enjoy and adjusting those activities as needed helps them stay engaged and find joy in their daily routines, making life better even with the challenges of Alzheimer's.

The Power of Pet Therapy

Pet therapy, also known as animal-assisted therapy, brings joy, comfort, and health benefits to people with Alzheimer's in ways that traditional therapies often can't. Imagine a room where tension melts into smiles and laughter, where the wag of a tail or the purr of a cat lifts spirits and reduces anxiety. This is the magic of pet therapy in Alzheimer's care. Research shows that interacting with animals can lower stress hormones like cortisol and boost endorphins, improving mood and emotional well-being. Plus, these interactions can encourage social engagement and physical activity, as people with Alzheimer's might walk a dog or pet a cat, supporting their physical health.

Choosing the right animal for pet therapy is important. Dogs and cats are common choices, but birds, fish, or rabbits can also be great companions. Dogs offer a comforting presence and can participate in activities like fetching or gentle walking, which helps with physical activity. Cats, with their soothing purrs and low-maintenance care, are perfect for those who need comfort without a lot of interaction. Birds, with their cheerful chirps and the routine care they require, offer companionship and a sense of purpose. Fish, with their graceful movements, are calming to watch. When selecting a pet, consider your loved one's past experiences and any allergies they might have. Make sure to choose an animal that is calm, gentle, and comfortable in different situations.

When introducing pet therapy, safety and comfort for both your loved one and the animal are key. Always supervise interactions to manage any unpredictable behaviors. Create a safe environment to prevent accidental harm, like scratching or biting. Regular health checks for the pet will help prevent the transmission of diseases. Also, consider the mobility and cognitive abilities of your loved one; a large, energetic dog might not be suitable for someone with balance or walking difficulties.

For caregivers who find full-time pet ownership daunting, there are alternatives. Many communities have organizations that offer pet therapy programs, bringing trained animals to visit people with Alzheimer's in their homes or care facilities. These visits provide the benefits of animal interaction without the responsibilities of daily care. Virtual pet interactions, like watching videos of animals, can also provide visual and auditory stimulation and evoke pleasant memories of past pets. Another option is creating a sensory garden that attracts local wildlife like birds or squirrels, providing a soothing connection to nature and a conversation starter.

Pet therapy offers a gentle yet powerful way to improve the lives of those with Alzheimer's. Through petting, caring for, or simply being near animals, people with Alzheimer's can find moments of joy and peace amidst the challenges of dementia, showing that sometimes, the best therapy comes on four legs with a dose of unconditional love.

Integrating Music and Art in Daily Care

Music and art therapy are powerful tools for helping people with Alzheimer's, providing joy and significant therapeutic benefits. Research shows that music therapy can reduce stress and anxiety, boost mood, and trigger memories from the past, offering people a connection to parts of themselves that seemed lost. Art therapy, meanwhile, allows for expression beyond words, giving people a way to communicate and connect when words fail them, and providing a tangible sense of accomplishment and pleasure.

When adding music therapy to daily routines, focus on personalization and enjoyment. Create playlists with songs that hold special meaning from your loved one's younger years. These familiar tunes can stir deep memories and emotions, often bringing comfort and moments of clarity. Encourage activities like singing along, clapping, or gently moving to the rhythm, which also provides mild physical exercise and boosts engagement. For example, if your loved one always enjoyed a particular band or genre, playing their songs during difficult times of the day can ease agitation and bring pleasure.

Art therapy can be included in home settings in various enriching and fulfilling ways. Start with simple, success-oriented projects to ensure the activity is enjoyable and not frustrating. Activities like finger painting, which don't require precise movements, or sculpting with clay, which can be soothing and tactile, are excellent choices. Use safe, non-toxic materials, and set up a comfortable space where they can create without constraints. The goal is not to produce a masterpiece but to engage in the act of creation, which can be a profoundly liberating and affirming experience for people with Alzheimer's.

Adapting these activities to suit the changing abilities of your loved one is imperative. As the disease progresses, lower the complexity of the tasks to make sure they remain doable and enjoyable. For music therapy, this might mean shifting from active participation in singing or dancing to simply listening to soothing melodies. In art therapy, moving from using fine brushes to broader strokes with sponges or creating collages with pre-cut pieces can help maintain the activity's accessibility and enjoyment.

By integrating music and art therapy into daily care, you not only enrich the day-to-day experiences of your loved one but also tap into the profound healing and communicative power of these therapies. They offer a way to connect, express, and remember, turning the caregiving environment into one of creativity, joy, and deep emotional engagement. These moments of connection, often filled with meaning, underscore the profound impact that thoughtful, personalized care can have on the quality of life for someone living with Alzheimer's.

Storytelling and Reminiscence Techniques

Reminiscence therapy is a warm and engaging approach that uses memories to brighten someone's day. Imagine sitting with your loved one, flipping through an old photo album, and seeing their eyes light up as they talk about past summer vacations or their first job. This is what reminiscence therapy is all about—a simple yet powerful way to connect with your loved one. By discussing past experiences and using prompts like photos, familiar objects, or music, you can help trigger memories and start meaningful conversations. This therapy taps into long-term memory, which often remains stronger than short-term memory in people with Alzheimer's, helping them feel more confident and connected as they recall their past.

When engaging in storytelling, your approach can make a big difference. Use simple, clear language—complex phrases or too many details can confuse rather than help. Encourage them to share stories from their past, but be ready to gently guide the conversation if they struggle with memory or get sidetracked. Asking open-ended questions can help keep the conversation going. For example, instead of asking if they remember their wedding day, say, "Tell me about your wedding day. What was it like?" This prompts a more detailed response instead of a simple 'yes' or 'no' answer.

Creating a reminiscence kit can deepen this experience. Gather items that are meaningful to the person—like a collection of favorite music, objects related to a hobby they enjoyed, or scents and textures tied to fond memories, such as a favorite perfume or fabric. These items serve as prompts to make recalling the past easier and more vivid. Notice which items evoke the strongest responses and use that information to guide future sessions. For instance, if a particular song always brings a smile, include music more often in your reminiscence activities.

The benefits of storytelling and reminiscence go beyond your loved one. As a caregiver, these sessions give you valuable insights into their life, helping you understand them better and connect on a personal level. These activities can also be incredibly rewarding, offering moments of joy and closeness that might be rare in daily interactions. They provide a low-stress way to engage and interact, which can be a welcome change from the more routine or challenging aspects of caregiving. Sharing these stories can turn a simple afternoon into a meaningful journey through their life, enriching your relationship and providing both of you with a sense of shared history and connection.

Physical Therapy and Exercise

Physical activity plays a pivotal role in Alzheimer's care, offering benefits that go beyond just physical health. Regular exercise can improve mobility, prevent muscle weakness, boost circulation, and may slow down the cognitive decline that comes with Alzheimer's disease. For caregivers, setting up and keeping a regular exercise routine can be a powerful way to manage the overall progression of the disease.

Physical therapy in Alzheimer's care focuses on creating exercise and movement plans tailored to your loved one's specific needs, which can change as the disease progresses. Professional physical therapists are trained to assess these needs and develop personalized exercise plans. These plans might focus on improving balance to prevent falls or include strength training to combat muscle weakness and maintain mobility. The goal is to keep the body as agile and functional as possible, which also helps support brain health.

At-home caregivers can integrate simple, safe exercises into the daily routine of your loved one. Some easy activities to consider are seated stretches, which are great for those with limited mobility and help maintain flexibility without the risk of falling. Gentle range-of-motion exercises, like arm raises or ankle rotations, can be done from a seated or standing position and are crucial for keeping joints flexible. For those who can, short walks around the home or in a nearby park can provide both physical exercise and sensory stimulation, which is important for mental health.

Encouraging regular physical activity can be challenging, especially if your loved one is resistant or uninterested. However, setting up a routine can be effective. Establish specific times each day for physical activity, making it a predictable part of the day that your loved one can get used to. Participating in these activities together can also make the experience more enjoyable and less of a chore. It's about making physical activity a shared, fun part of the day, which can significantly increase the willingness to participate.

Through these strategies—professional physical therapy tailored to individual needs, simple home exercises to maintain physical health, and a routine that includes regular physical activity—you can help manage the symptoms of Alzheimer's effectively. This proactive approach not only maintains physical health but also contributes to overall well-being, offering a more balanced and holistic approach to managing the disease.

Each step you take, no matter how small, brings you closer to improving the well-being of your loved one. These activities are not just about keeping the body active; they're about enriching lives, providing structure, support, and a sense of accomplishment.

Innovative Caregiving Techniques From Around the Globe

Around the globe, Alzheimer's care is approached in diverse ways, influenced by various cultures and healthcare philosophies. By examining these different perspectives, we might discover valuable practices to incorporate into our own care routines. Below, we'll look at how different cultures address the challenges of Alzheimer's care and uncover lessons we can apply at home.

Europe

In many parts of Europe, particularly the Netherlands, you'll find an innovative concept known as dementia villages. These specially designed communities offer a secure, village-like environment where people with dementia can live, socialize, and receive care while maintaining a high level of independence. Everything within the village, from grocery stores to cinemas, is structured to allow residents to engage in everyday activities safely and comfortably.

This approach to Alzheimer's care emphasizes a familiar, engaging lifestyle, helping to preserve residents' skills and reduce the stress and confusion often associated with traditional care settings. Family caregivers may want to take notes, as this method highlights the benefits of creating a familiar and engaging environment at home. Activities like maintaining a small garden together or setting up a home-based shop can allow people with Alzheimer's to continue to enjoy their favorite hobbies and pastimes.

Asia

In Asian countries like China and Japan, the approach to Alzheimer's care often centers around family-focused care. Here, family piety and obligation play significant roles in caregiving. Multi-generational living arrangements are common, so caregiving responsibilities are shared among family members.

This integrated approach provides strong support and continuous care, which is vital as the needs of a person with Alzheimer's grows. For those in more individualistic cultures, the lesson might be to foster stronger family ties by involving multiple family members in caregiving, sharing responsibilities, and supporting each other through regular family meetings to discuss care strategies and emotional challenges.

Africa

In Africa, community-based models of care are prevalent. The extended community often takes on the role of caring for its elderly members, including those with Alzheimer's. This communal responsibility can alleviate pressure on individual caregivers and foster a sense of belonging and purpose. Community centers often act as hubs where elders can engage in social activities, keeping their minds active and spirits high.

This model highlights the importance of social engagement and community support in Alzheimer's care—something that can be replicated by connecting with local Alzheimer's associations, joining support groups, and participating in community activities.

Inspired by dementia villages, Amelia made some changes at home for her grandmother, Ruby, who has Alzheimer's. She turned their backyard into a garden with walking paths and set up a "shop" in the living room, where Ruby loved arranging items like she used to in her antiques store. Amelia also started holding family dinners on Sundays to discuss Ruby's care. Everyone pitched in; her brother Hudson took over groceries, and her sister Caroline took Ruby to the park. This brought the family closer together. Amelia also joined a local Alzheimer's support group, which offered social activities like art classes and music therapy that kept Ruby engaged and happy. These simple changes brought joy to Ruby's life and gave Amelia the support she needed.

Adapting caregiving strategies to fit your unique situation involves a blend of creativity and practicality. If the idea of a dementia village intrigues you, consider creating a simplified version in your home or neighborhood. Could you set up safe, walkable paths in your garden? Or, maybe you could collaborate with neighbors to create a safe community space where your loved one feels free to roam. Using a family-focused model often involves having conversations with your family about how everyone can contribute, whether it's through direct care or providing respite for primary caregivers.

Incorporating diverse caregiving strategies can break the monotony of daily routines and introduce fresh perspectives that reinvigorate your approach to care. These varied strategies can improve the care you provide by offering new ways to engage your loved one. They can also reduce your stress by sharing the load and, most importantly, improve the overall well-being of your loved one by keeping them integrated into a community.

Remember, every small change or new approach can make a significant difference in the life of your loved one. Whether you adopt elements of a dementia village, give family-focused care a try, or integrate community-based models, there are numerous ideas waiting to be tailored to the needs of you and your loved one.

Make a Difference with Your Review
Unlock the Secret of Compassionate Care

"Individually, we are one drop. Together, we are an ocean."

— *Ryunosuke Satoro*

Taking care of someone is one of the most generous things we can do. Your compassion makes the world a better place. Now, you have the opportunity to make an even bigger impact by helping others on their caregiving journey!

Are you ready to help someone like you—someone who's navigating the ups and downs of caring for a loved one with Alzheimer's?

My mission is to make understanding and caring for those with Alzheimer's easier and more fulfilling for everyone. But to reach more people who need this guide, I need your help.

Most people choose their next read based on reviews. Your thoughts could guide another caregiver just starting their journey. Your review could help...

- one more caregiver find comfort knowing they're not alone.
- one more family discover better ways to connect with their loved one.
- one more friend feel confident to offer support.
- one more person find hope in the face of burnout and overwhelm.
- one more heart feel understood.

Leaving a review costs nothing, but your words could make a world of difference to someone who needs this support.

To help, simply scan the QR code below to share your review:

From the bottom of my heart, thank you for being part of this journey! Your compassion, words, and care are helping change lives.

Renée Remy

Section Four
Navigating the Caregiver's Emotional Journey

Sydney had had a difficult day of caregiving. Her aunt Cindy had been upset with the false belief that her favorite pair of reading glasses had been stolen by the private caregiver and kept yelling at the caregiver. Cindy refused to calm down because the caregiver would not give Cindy back her glasses and denied taking them. Sydney listened to her aunt's concerns and validated Cindy's emotions. Once Cindy felt heard and calmed down, Sydney encouraged Cindy to do some gardening with the caregiver. Sydney had found the glasses, returned them to Cindy, and the three of them celebrated the return of the glasses. Then Cindy sat down to watch a nature show on TV. Sydney took a few deep breaths, expressed gratitude that she was able to de-escalate the situation and even find the glasses. Then she celebrated with a smile and took a break while Cindy was occupied.

This moment is yours—precious and hard-earned. It's in these quiet times that the weight of caregiving can truly be felt, both in its demands and its profound importance. In this chapter, we'll discuss how to recognize signs of burnout, establish self-care routines, and set boundaries to protect your well-being.

Recognizing and Managing Burnout

As a caregiver, it's easy to become so focused on someone else's well-being that you miss the early signs of your own burnout. Burnout can sneak up quietly, manifesting as constant fatigue, a feeling of detachment, or frustration over small things. It's more than just being tired; burnout makes you feel emotionally and physically drained, leading to deeper feelings of depression and irritability. Everyday can start to feel like an uphill battle. Recognizing these signs early is vital for both your well-being and the quality of care you offer.

To tackle burnout, it's essential to establish a solid self-care routine. Think of self-care as your lifeboat during stormy times—it keeps you afloat and helps you stay resilient. Start with regular physical activities, like a morning walk or a yoga session during breaks, to boost your physical and mental energy. Also, prioritize sleep by maintaining a consistent sleep schedule and creating a bedtime routine that helps you unwind, such as reading or meditating. A 15 to 30 minute meditation in the morning can provide you with more resilience for the challenges of the day ahead. If your loved one often wakes you during the night, try to take a naps when possible, or make time for a 10 to 15 minute meditation during the day to re-energize your body.

Nutrition also plays a big role in preventing burnout. A balanced diet keeps your energy levels steady throughout the day. Include plenty of fruits, vegetables, lean proteins, and whole grains in your meals. And don't forget to drink enough water! On the emotional front, mindfulness and deep-breathing exercises can help manage stress. Spend a few minutes each day meditating or doing deep-breathing exercises to center your thoughts and clear your mind.

Sometimes, though, self-care might not be enough. If you feel overwhelmed or notice persistent symptoms of depression or anxiety, reaching out to a counselor or joining a support group can help. These resources offer professional insights and empathetic understanding from those who've been through similar experiences. They remind you that you're not alone, providing both comfort and practical strategies to manage the challenges you face.

Setting boundaries can also help prevent overcommitment. It's okay to say no or to delegate tasks to others. Communicate openly with family members or other caregivers about your limits, and don't hesitate to ask for help when you need it. Setting boundaries isn't a sign of weakness but a smart move to ensure you can keep caring effectively. It prevents resentment and keeps your relationship with your loved one positive and strong.

By recognizing the signs of burnout early, actively engaging in self-care, seeking help when needed, and setting clear boundaries, you can protect your well-being. This approach not only improves your caregiving skills but also allows you to be there for your loved one in the ways that truly matter. It's about finding balance, caring for yourself, and embracing the role of caregiver with renewed strength and compassion.

How to Deal with Guilt and Grief

When you're deeply involved in caring for someone, it's normal to feel guilt and grief, especially when it's your loved one who has Alzheimer's. These feelings can be intense and complicated. You might feel guilty for thinking you're not doing enough or for the tough decisions you make about their care. You might also feel bad for getting frustrated, losing your patience, or thinking about taking a break. Understanding that these feelings are normal is the first step to handling them.

Guilt often comes from having high expectations for yourself and wanting to provide the best care possible. There's a difference between irrational guilt, which is baseless and overwhelming, and constructive guilt, which can help you improve your caregiving. Understanding this distinction is important. For example, feeling guilty for losing patience can lead you to find better ways to manage stress. To deal with this, acknowledge your feelings without judging yourself, understand what triggers them, and talk to someone who can offer a different perspective, like another caregiver or a counselor.

This can be very relieving and help you realize these feelings are a common response to a tough role.

> *One afternoon, after a series of particularly tough days, Imani decided to take a short break and sit in the backyard with a book while her husband, Malik, was napping. She had only been outside for a few minutes when she heard Malik calling for her in a panic. Imani rushed back inside to find him confused and upset, unable to understand why she wasn't there. She felt a surge of guilt for leaving him alone, even briefly. That evening, overwhelmed by guilt, Imani shared her experience with a close friend. Her friend listened empathetically and reassured her that taking breaks is essential to her well-being and doesn't make her a bad caregiver. Imani was reminded that she couldn't pour from an empty cup, and moving forward, she put a baby monitor inside to keep an ear on Malik when she needed time to herself.*

Talking openly with friends or family can help you cope with guilt. They can reassure you that you're doing your best, or they might share their own experiences, reminding you that you're not alone. Practicing self-forgiveness is crucial. Remember, no caregiver is perfect, and it's okay to have weak moments. Focus on what you do right and celebrate small successes. Keeping a journal where you note positive moments in caregiving—times when you felt connected or when a care strategy worked well—can boost your morale and reduce guilt.

Grief is also a significant challenge in caregiving. You may grieve for the person your loved one used to be while continuing to care for who they are now. This type of grief, known as anticipatory grief, is complex because you're mourning someone who is still physically present. You may experience many emotions, including sadness, anger, denial, and even relief. Understanding the process and different aspects of grief can help you recognize and accept your feelings. It's important to let yourself feel these emotions rather than pushing them away, as processing them is vital for your emotional health.

Sometimes, guilt and grief can feel overwhelming. Talking to a therapist or counselor who specializes in caregiver support can be very helpful. They can offer strategies tailored to your situation, helping you manage your emotions effectively. They provide a safe space to express and work through your feelings, which can be very validating and healing. Also, joining a caregiver support group can connect you with others in similar situations. Sharing your experiences and hearing others' stories can offer comfort and practical advice on coping with the emotional ups and downs of caregiving.

Remember, dealing with guilt and grief isn't about eliminating these feelings; it's about managing them, so they don't take over your life. By acknowledging these emotions, seeking support, and practicing self-care, you can handle these complex feelings better while continuing to provide compassionate care.

Building Emotional Strength

Think of emotional strength as a skill that improves with practice. Every day as a caregiver brings new challenges, and each challenge is an opportunity to adapt and grow. At the end of a tough day, take a moment to reflect on what went well and what could have been handled differently. Did an unexpected outburst catch you off guard? Think about what might have triggered it and how you might respond differently next time. This reflection isn't just about solving problems; it's about finding positive aspects in difficult situations, which can lead to a more hopeful outlook and better outcomes in the future.

Building a supportive network is crucial. This network should include friends, family, community resources, and fellow caregivers who understand what you're going through. These connections can offer both practical advice and emotional support. Join support groups, either in person or online. These groups can be a lifeline on tough days, providing encouragement and understanding from people who really get the nuances of Alzheimer's care. They remind you that you're not alone and that others have faced similar challenges and found ways to manage them.

As you practice the techniques listed in this chapter, you will discover that these 3 C's will enhance each one in helping you build emotional strength:

1. **(Be) Conscious.** Reflect on each day and become more aware, or conscious of the circumstances, your thoughts, and your reactions for both things that went well and things that could have gone better. This awareness will guide your future responses and decisions moving forward.
2. **Celebrate.** Celebrate what you noticed. Celebrate things that went well. Celebrate what you discovered during your reflection for ways to make a future challenge better. Celebrate that you simply got through another day.
3. **Connect.** Engage your support network: unload your burdens, ask for advice, share your wins, have fun, laugh.

Regular reflection can be a powerful tool for building resilience. It helps you process your experiences, celebrate your successes, and learn from challenges. Consider keeping a journal to write down your thoughts and feelings about your caregiving experiences. Writing can be very therapeutic, helping you to process complex emotions and stress in a constructive way. It's also a great way to track your growth over time, showing you how far you've come and reminding you of the positive impact you're having on your loved one's life.

Another way to reflect is to create voice recordings - which can even be done on your cell phone, computer apps, and stand-alone devices. If you are creative, you can reflect by creating mind maps, a sketchbook journal, or by writing a song. Regardless of how you record your reflections, there is power in taking it out of your head and putting it in another format that you can review later.

Take the time to review your successes once a month and celebrate them. Celebration can be as simple as a knowing smile or doing a happy dance. Celebrating your successes both in the moment and upon monthly reflection releases three hormones: dopamine, endorphins, and serotonin. These hormones lower anxiety and increase a feeling of happiness. Since your body feels good when you celebrate, your mind will start to support your efforts to find more reasons to celebrate, and you'll feel more resilient.

Participating in caregiver support group discussions can also help build resilience. These discussions often highlight common issues and different perspectives on handling caregiving challenges. They can provide validation and new insights, helping you see your situation in a new light and benefit from others' experiences. This can reinforce your resilience by integrating new coping strategies and perspectives into your approach.

Maintaining hobbies and interests outside of caregiving is essential for resilience. These activities can provide a much-needed break, a sense of normalcy and joy. They remind you of your identity beyond being a caregiver. Whether it's gardening, painting, hiking, or reading, these activities can rejuvenate your spirit and reduce stress. They're not just hobbies; they're part of your self-care routine, helping you maintain your emotional health and overall well-being.

By nurturing these aspects of resilience—learning from each day, building a supportive community, reflecting regularly, and maintaining your own interests—you equip yourself to handle the emotional demands of caregiving. This doesn't just benefit you; it directly improves the care and support you can provide for your loved one, making each day a little easier and a lot more fulfilling.

Stress Reduction Techniques

Resilience is often seen as the ability to bounce back from difficulties, but for caregivers, it's more like being a strong tree that bends in the wind but stays firmly rooted. Building resilience as a caregiver isn't about returning to how things were—because each day brings new challenges with your loved one's condition changing constantly. Instead, it's about improving your ability to handle stress and setbacks gracefully, gaining insights from each experience, and becoming stronger and more adaptable.

When you're caring for someone with Alzheimer's, finding moments to breathe deeply and relax might seem impossible. Yet, these moments are essential, not just for your well-being but also for maintaining the endurance you need to care for someone with Alzheimer's. Here are some effective relaxation techniques that can help ease the stress that often comes with your role as a caregiver:

- **Deep Breathing Exercises:** Deep breathing exercises are a simple yet powerful tool to reduce stress. Inhale slowly through your nose, allowing your chest and lower belly to rise. Hold the breath for a moment, then exhale slowly through your mouth. Repeating this exercise for a few minutes can activate your body's natural relaxation response, significantly reducing tension and anxiety.
- **Progressive Muscle Relaxation:** Progressive muscle relaxation involves tensing and then relaxing each muscle group in your body to reduce physical tension. Start from your toes and work your way up to your head, tensing each muscle group, holding the tension, and then releasing it. Visualize the stress melting away as you release the tension, helping you become more aware of when you are physically holding stress.

- **Mindfulness:** Known for reducing stress and improving mental health, mindfulness involves staying present in the moment and observing your thoughts without judgment. Practice mindfulness anytime, anywhere—while washing dishes, walking, or sitting quietly—by focusing on the present moment and letting thoughts pass without attachment. This helps maintain a clearer mind and reduces overwhelming feelings.
- **Brain Breaks:** This technique gives the brain a break from the constant stream of thoughts and negative emotions. Concentrate on a single sensation (touch, sound, smell, taste, sight) or your breathing for at least 10-30 seconds. For example, listen to the sounds furthest away for 15 seconds, then switch to the closest sounds for another 15 seconds. This mindfulness break resets your brain and immediately brings more peace and calm. You can do this while preparing a meal, changing a diaper, or dealing with a difficult situation.
- **Morning Meditation:** Morning meditation can result in a peace and calm that stays with you for quite a while. Work your way up from 5 to 30 minutes of meditation before you start your day. This practice creates a foundation of emotional stability, increasing your resilience and giving you more strength to handle daily challenges.
- **Technology**: Stress management and relaxation apps offer guided meditations, soothing sounds, and relaxation exercises to help you unwind after a long day. Spending a few minutes with these apps can lower your stress levels and make you feel refreshed and ready to face the challenges of caregiving again.

Incorporating these relaxation techniques can make a significant difference in your daily routine, but it's not the only strategy that can improve your well-being.

> *I enjoy a morning meditation before I get out of bed. I imagine myself being held in a warm, glowing light that provides comfort and support, and I smile as I sink into this place of total love and peace. When my mind wanders (as it always does), I gently bring my focus back to this nourishing place. I usually set a timer before I start, in case I fall asleep. Once I am fully immersed, I feel comfortably warmer and express my gratitude for the unconditional love I am feeling. If the timer goes off first, I turn it off and return to my meditation long enough to express gratitude and then end with a smile. Ending with a smile helps extend the feeling of relaxation and peace. The more you practice, the faster you can enter this space.*

Exercise is also important for both your mind and body. Regular physical activity can boost your mood, enhance your energy levels, and reduce stress. Simple activities like walking or stretching can easily fit into your day and allow you to keep your loved one involved as well. For example, if your loved one uses a wheelchair, taking a daily walk around the block can be refreshing for both of you.

Incorporating stretching exercises can also be a great way to stay active. Gentle yoga sessions in the morning or before bed can help maintain physical flexibility and mental wellness. These exercises don't need to be long or intense; even short sessions can make a big difference. There are also many online resources and apps that offer guided yoga sessions for all skill levels and ages, making it easy to find a routine that works for you.

Maintaining social connections and hobbies might seem tough when your schedule is packed with caregiving tasks, but they are key to relieving stress. Rediscover activities you enjoy, whether it's painting, gardening, or playing a musical instrument. These hobbies are not just ways to relax; they are ways to express yourself and find joy.

If you're ever concerned about your health, don't hesitate to see a doctor. Sometimes the stress and worry of thinking something is wrong can make you feel worse. Take the time to find out if there is something physically wrong with you – don't wait and neglect yourself until it's too late. According to a study, 40-60% of caregivers die before the people they're caring for, and most of these individuals are caring for loved ones with Alzheimer's. Why? A lack of self-care. Taking care of yourself is not optional, but essential.

Sometimes the strategies we use on our own aren't enough to handle stress effectively. In these cases, seeking professional support is a smart step toward maintaining your mental health. Therapists or counselors who specialize in caregiver support can offer valuable guidance and tools for managing stress. They provide a safe space to express and process your feelings, helping you develop strategies to handle the emotional demands of caregiving. Remember, seeking help is a sign of strength, not weakness. It shows your commitment to your well-being and the quality of care you're providing to your loved one.

By incorporating these stress-reduction techniques into your life, you can create a more balanced approach to caregiving, one that includes time for self-care and emotional well-being. These practices not only help in managing day-to-day stresses but also make you more resilient, enabling you to provide the best care possible while also taking care of yourself.

Embracing Change and New Normals

Caring for someone with Alzheimer's means constantly adapting to a 'new normal.' This isn't a single adjustment, but an ongoing process of changes in your loved one's abilities, personality, and needs. Welcoming these changes isn't about losing hope or love; it's about reshaping your expectations and finding new ways to provide the best care possible. It requires an open heart and a flexible mindset as the person you care for gradually changes from who they once were.

Adapting to this new normal starts with acceptance. Acceptance doesn't mean giving up; it's about acknowledging the reality of the situation without feeling hopeless or judgmental. This can be really hard, especially when you see significant declines in their memory or personality. You might find your loved one forgetting cherished memories or struggling with simple tasks they used to do easily. Adapting your care might mean simplifying communication, modifying daily activities to match their abilities, or creating new routines that bring comfort and structure. It also means being alert and responsive to their changing needs, which can vary daily.

Staying flexible in your caregiving is crucial. What works today might not work tomorrow, and what fails one day might work the next. This unpredictable situation requires you to be observant, creative, and patient. For example, if a certain activity or routine brings them comfort, try to include it more in your day, but be ready to change if it stops working. As symptoms evolve, your strategies will need to change too. This might involve using new tools to help with memory, like reminder apps or memory books, or adjusting the home to make it safer and easier to move around.

If change is not something that you relish, consider comparing it to something you do enjoy. For example, you can think of it as a science experiment where you're trying to find out the properties of this new and interesting substance called Alzheimer's. You take notes as you notice the positive effects and change experiments as the results change. Or you can think of yourself as an explorer in a foreign land, with new and interesting changes around every corner and sometimes every day. You have the opportunity to learn new ways of communicating and new customs for behaving as you journey through the land of Alzheimer's. So how can you find the curiosity and exploration in the journey? Is it like growing a garden, playing a video game, or maybe painting a picture with an ever-changing landscape? You get to decide.

Celebrating the journey means recognizing and appreciating every step of the caregiving experience. Despite the hardships, there are moments of joy, connection, and triumph to be found. It might be a shared laugh over a meal, successfully trying a new care strategy, or a peaceful afternoon spent together. These moments are worth celebrating and can be deeply affirming. They remind you why you've taken on this role and highlight the deep, enduring connection you have with your loved one. Celebrating these successes with family and friends can also strengthen your support network, uplifting everyone involved and reinforcing the bonds that sustain you all.

In welcoming this new normal, remember that change is not just about loss. It's also about adaptation, growth, and the deep love that guides your journey as a caregiver. Each day brings new challenges but also new opportunities to connect, grow, and make meaningful contributions to the life of someone you care about deeply. In this ever-changing environment, your flexibility, resilience, and compassionate heart are your greatest assets.

Setting Realistic Expectations and Goals

When you first become a caregiver, it's like starting a journey that will change many times along the way. Setting realistic goals and expectations is crucial for navigating this path effectively. It involves understanding the progressive nature of Alzheimer's and adjusting your goals as the disease progresses. At first, your goals might focus on maintaining as much independence as possible, like managing personal hygiene or participating in social activities. As the disease progresses, these goals may shift toward ensuring comfort and quality interactions, such as holding hands and enjoying a sunny day on the porch.

As you gain more experience and knowledge, you'll also need to reassess your expectations. You'll develop a deeper understanding of the disease, the specific reactions of your loved one, and your own capacity as a caregiver. This learning curve allows you to continually refine your strategies and expectations. For instance, while you might initially hope to handle all caregiving tasks on your own, you may realize that seeking help from professional caregivers or community resources is not only reasonable but necessary. Adjusting your expectations can help prevent feelings of failure and frustration that come from unrealistic goals.

Balancing optimism with practicality is another core aspect of setting goals in Alzheimer's care. It's good to hope for the best outcomes from your care strategies and treatments, but also to be prepared for the gradual decline that comes with the disease. This balance helps you stay proactive rather than reactive. For example, while you might be optimistic about the benefits of a new medication or therapy, being practical about the gradual progression of the disease will prepare you for changes in your loved one's condition.

Acknowledging and celebrating small victories is essential on this journey. These moments offer a respite from the challenges and are key for emotional reward and motivation. Perhaps your loved one remembers a detail from their past during a reminiscence therapy session, or they show a moment of clarity where they recognize you and express affection. These instances, though small, are significant. They remind you that your efforts are making a difference in their quality of life, bringing joy and satisfaction to both of you. Celebrating these achievements can uplift your spirits and encourage you to continue caregiving with renewed energy and hope.

Setting realistic goals and expectations creates a framework that guides your caregiving. This framework helps in providing the best possible care and supports your emotional well-being by aligning your efforts with achievable outcomes. It's about finding satisfaction in what you can do, rather than disappointment in what is beyond anyone's control. With each small victory, you build an array of positive experiences that enrich both your life and that of your loved one, making every day a meaningful part of your shared journey.

Coping With Unexpected Challenges

When you're in the thick of caregiving, unexpected challenges can hit like sudden storms, disrupting your routine and demanding immediate action. Maybe your loved one becomes agitated or aggressive, a new health issue arises, or the home care assistant calls in sick at the last minute. These moments test your resilience and adaptability, requiring quick thinking and flexible responses.

The first step in managing these surprises is to anticipate them as much as possible. While you can't predict everything, having a general plan for unexpected behaviors or medical emergencies can reduce panic and allow for more controlled responses. For example, if sudden behavioral changes occur, having a calm-down kit ready— with soothing music, a favorite blanket, or a photo album—can help. For medical emergencies, keep an up-to-date list of medications, allergies, and doctor contacts. This list should be easily accessible on your phone or kept in a visible place at home.

Being flexible is crucial. This might mean having a backup plan for care when regular support isn't available. Connect with more than one caregiving agency or have a list of friends or family members who can step in when needed. Consider taking basic health emergency courses, like CPR or first aid, to give you the confidence to handle sudden health issues until professional help arrives.

The emotional toll of dealing with these sudden challenges can be heavy. Developing strong emotional coping techniques is as important as managing the practical aspects of caregiving. Practices like deep breathing exercises or mindfulness can help center your thoughts and reduce anxiety during high-stress situations. Keeping a journal can also be a therapeutic way to process stress after the event, allowing you to reflect on what happened and how you handled it. This reflection is not just about assessing, but also acknowledging the effort you put in and the care you gave, which can be emotionally uplifting.

Viewing each unexpected challenge as a learning opportunity can really change how you approach caregiving. After dealing with a sudden issue, take a moment to think about what worked and what didn't. Could you have done anything differently? Were there resources you could have used better? Writing down these incidents and your thoughts about them can be very helpful for future situations. This not only prepares you better but also helps you understand and improve your caregiving skills. Over time, this knowledge makes your caregiving practice more resilient, allowing you to handle new challenges with more confidence and ability.

Time Management Tips

Caring for someone with Alzheimer's often feels like there aren't enough hours in the day. With managing medications, appointments, daily tasks, and unexpected situations, time becomes a precious resource. Here's how you can make the most of your time, prioritize what truly needs your attention, and carve out those much-needed moments of rest.

Start by learning how to prioritize and delegate tasks by understanding what needs to be done immediately and what can wait. For example, giving medication and preparing meals are time-sensitive, while organizing the closet can wait. Use daily lists to keep track of tasks and mark them off as you go, which can also give you a sense of accomplishment. Delegation is your friend. You don't have to do everything yourself. Family members, friends, or professional caregivers can share the load. Maybe a neighbor can pick up groceries for you, or a family member can sit with your loved one while you take a break. It's about working smarter, not harder, to ensure that all necessary care is provided without wearing yourself out.

Using organizational tools can significantly improve your efficiency. Digital calendars are great for keeping track of medical appointments, social visits, and daily tasks. Set reminders for everything from doctor's appointments to time for your own lunch. Apps designed specifically for caregivers can help you track tasks, log health information, and even coordinate care among family members and professional helpers. Don't overlook the value of traditional tools like planners or wall calendars which can be more accessible and continually in view for quick reference.

There are many smartphone apps designed specifically to help manage Alzheimer's care. Apps like 'CareZone' let you store health information, schedule medication reminders, and track doctor appointments all in one place.

Setting realistic goals each day can help you manage your time better. Understand that some days will be more productive than others, and that's okay. Your goals need to be flexible, reflecting the changing needs of your loved one. If you set daily and weekly goals, make sure they're achievable and allow room for the unexpected. Additionally, know your limits. Recognize when your plate is full and resist the urge to take on more tasks than you can handle. Overcommitment can lead to stress and burnout, which helps neither you nor the person you care for.

Finding time for breaks is not a luxury—it's necessary for your well-being and effectiveness as a caregiver. Regular breaks help prevent fatigue and keep your spirits up. Coordinate with other family members or caregivers to schedule these pauses. You might use this time for a walk, a nap, reading, or another relaxing activity. Consider respite care services, which can provide short-term breaks for caregivers. Participating in caregiver support groups can also offer structured break times where you engage with others who understand your experiences and can offer support and advice. These breaks are not just gaps in your schedule; they are vital moments that recharge your energy and focus, enabling you to care for your loved one with renewed patience and love.

By mastering these strategies, you can create a balanced schedule that meets both your needs and those of your loved one, making each day more manageable and less stressful. Remember, effective time management in caregiving isn't just about making it through the day; it's about making the day meaningful, providing quality care for your loved one while also taking care of yourself.

Finding and Engaging with Support Groups

Finding the right support group can sometimes feel like trying to find a light in the fog. You know it's there, and you know it'll be helpful, but how do you find it? When I first started looking for support groups for Alzheimer's caregivers, I felt completely overwhelmed. There were so many options, but which one would be a good fit for me? If you're feeling the same way, don't worry—you're not alone. There are plenty of resources to help you connect with others who understand what you're going through, and the best way to start is simply to join one and see how it goes. As you connect with others, you can even ask them what other groups they might recommend. In some cities, the best support groups are found by word of mouth.

Where to Start:

- **Your Local Alzheimer's Association Chapter:** They often have a list of active support groups in your area and can point you in the right direction. Some of these groups focus on things like general caregiving tips, while others might concentrate on legal advice or emotional support. It can be helpful to reach out to multiple groups to find the one that suits you best.
- **The Internet:** There are plenty of online platforms and social media groups where caregivers from all over the globe come together to connect, ask questions, and share stories and advice. Platforms like Facebook have dedicated groups and forums for Alzheimer's care. You can see how active social media groups are by seeing how many posts have been added in the last 1-2 weeks. You'll want to start with a group that appears to be active. You can also find groups that meet virtually, which can be useful if you can't leave home due to your caregiving responsibilities.
- **Other Options:** Here are some additional options for finding a support group that fits your needs. These businesses, people, and resources often have information on support groups where you can meet with other caregivers face-to-face:

  ○ Faith-based organizations
  ○ Community centers
  ○ Senior centers
  ○ Libraries

- ○ Meetup.com
- ○ Hospitals
- ○ The National Association of Area Agencies on Aging
- ○ Your doctor's office
- ○ Local mental health professionals
- ○ The National Institute on Aging (NIA)

The educational resources available on various online platforms can also be particularly helpful. These platforms offer tutorials, live webinars, and guides on Alzheimer's care, helping you stay informed about the latest care techniques and research.

Joining a support group offers more than just practical caregiving tips. These groups give you a place to share your experiences and feelings without judgment. Talking with others who understand the unique challenges you're facing can give you a different perspective and insight into new coping strategies. You might even hear about solutions you hadn't considered or heard about before. It's incredibly comforting and reassuring to speak with people who truly get what you're going through. The emotional support you receive can lead to less stress and a stronger sense of community, making you feel less alone in your journey.

Blake was overwhelmed managing his father's Alzheimer's care. Juggling work, raising his three kids as a single father, and his dad's increasing needs left him exhausted. A nurse suggested joining a support group, and Blake found one through the local Alzheimer's Association. At the first meeting, he was warmly welcomed and immediately felt at ease. Hearing others share similar struggles made him realize he wasn't alone. The group offered helpful advice, like using a whiteboard to track daily tasks and finding local respite care. Over time, these meetings became Blake's sanctuary, offering emotional support and practical tips that made him feel more confident and less alone. This support network improved both his and his father's daily life, as well as his family's, making everything a bit more manageable. Blake noted that oddly enough, attending the support group seemed to give him more time and energy, as he became more emotionally resilient and efficient.

If you find a support group you'd like to join, here's how to make the most of your time:

1. **Be an Active Participant:** Share your experiences and insights, ask questions, and offer support to others. Being active helps build a sense of community and makes the experience much more rewarding.
2. **Show Up Consistently:** Regular attendance is key. It helps you build lasting relationships and stay up-to-date with discussions and resources. These connections can become your lifeline, offering support and understanding when you need it most.
3. **Be Vulnerable:** Share your true feelings and challenges. Honesty allows you to get the most relevant advice and support from the group. It also builds trust within the group and encourages other people to be more open in response to your step of courage.
4. **Respect Confidentiality:** Keep group discussions private to build trust and make everyone feel safe sharing their experiences.
5. **Set Goals:** Think about what you want to get out of the group and actively work toward these goals. Maybe you're there to become a better caregiver, or perhaps you're trying to take better care of your mental health.

By following these tips, you can make the most of your support group experience and find the encouragement and understanding you need on your caregiving journey.

But what if there's no group nearby, or if existing groups don't quite meet your needs? Starting your own support group can be a great way to meet your specific needs and help others. Find a meeting place like a community center, library, local cafe, or even start one virtually. Promote your group through community boards, social media, and local clinics. For the first meeting, prepare a simple agenda including a meet-and-greet, discussing members' goals, and planning future meetings. Managing a support group can deepen your understanding of Alzheimer's care while building a supportive community.

The Benefits of Professional Caregiving Services

C onsidering professional Alzheimer's caregiving services might feel overwhelming, but it opens new and beneficial opportunities for both you and your loved one. These services come in different forms, such as in-home care, adult day care centers, and full-time residential care facilities. Each option has its own benefits, designed to meet the different stages of the disease and the needs of both your loved one and your family.

In-home care agencies and private caregivers can be particularly beneficial as they allow your loved one to stay in the comfort of their own home while getting the help they need. This might include assistance with daily activities, managing medications, and even medical nursing services. Adult day care centers offer social activities and therapies that keep your loved one engaged and active, which can help slow the progression of the disease. For more advanced stages, full-time residential care facilities provide around-the-clock care, making sure all medical and daily needs are met in a safe environment.

Blending professional care with family caregiving can be challenging, but it can also increase the amount of support your loved one has.

Open communication is key, so be sure to establish a clear and consistent way to interact with the professionals responsible for your loved one's care. This helps ensure that your loved one's needs and preferences are met. Regular meetings or updates can help keep everyone on the same page, contributing to a smooth and continuous care experience.

Choosing the right service requires some thought. When looking at facilities, start by looking at the staff's qualifications and training to make sure they have experience with Alzheimer's care. A lower staff-to-patient ratio often means more personalized attention, which is crucial for those who might wander or need more assistance. Cleanliness and safety are must-haves, as they directly impact the well-being of your loved one. Listening to the experiences of other families whose loved ones have entered these facilities can provide valuable insights into the quality of care and their satisfaction with the services provided.

For in-home caregiving services, begin by making a list of your specific needs. Consider the following:

- Number of days per week you would like
- Number of hours per day and times of day you prefer
- Specific housekeeping duties to be completed (e.g. laundry, cleaning bathroom and kitchen after use, vacuuming, sweeping, watering plants)
- Meal prep and feeding
- Incontinent care
- Personal daily hygiene care
- Medication management
- Languages you would like them to speak
- Spiritual or religious backgrounds
- Willingness to engage your loved one in activities like drawing or going for walks

- Chauffeuring your loved one
- Ability to work with pets in the home

Caregiving agencies and private caregivers both have their pros and cons. Caregiving agencies promise that they have confirmed the caregiver's background and skills. They also take care of all government regulations for having an in-home caregiver. Private caregivers may cost less due to not having to pay the agency overhead and be willing to do more household chores, but you become responsible for background checks and tax and legal requirements for your state.

The decision to seek professional help might bring up feelings of guilt or apprehension. You may feel like you're passing off your responsibilities to someone else or worry about how your loved one will adapt to new caregivers. It's important to remember that using professional services doesn't mean you care any less. Rather, it's a proactive step to provide the best care for your loved one while also taking care of yourself.

Professional caregiving services can help prevent burnout, allowing you to stay strong, present, and effective as a caregiver. By seeing professional care as a positive addition to your own loving care, you can reduce your emotional burden. This can help you focus more on spending quality time with your loved one rather than stressing about daily care responsibilities.

Section Five
Legal and Financial Planning

Muffet learned, after caring for her mother through an illness, how important it is to have legal documents like a Trust and designated health and financial decision-makers in place. Her mother had discussed these plans with her and her brother long before they needed to take action, making the decisions for her mother's care much easier. If Muffet and her brother ever faced disagreements, they turned to their mother's documented wishes to guide their decisions. Her mother's foresight was a beacon during some of the most challenging moments of the caregiving journey, preserving family relationships. Inspired by this, Muffet quickly ensured that all her own plans were in place, understanding how important it was. To her, these plans weren't just documents—they were a love letter to her family, offering them peace of mind for the future.

Anyone who has been on this journey will tell you just how important it is to handle legal and financial planning matters as soon as possible. As daunting as it may seem, setting up the right legal safeguards is an act of love and foresight. It ensures that even as your loved one's ability to make decisions diminishes, their dignity, preferences, and welfare are upheld, especially during family disagreements. In moments of uncertainty, you'll have guidance on the decisions that need to be made, and you can move forward guilt-free, knowing you did your best.

Some people find starting this process rather scary or daunting because they don't understand all the legal mumbo jumbo and financial language. The intention of this chapter is to make some of the key terms, forms, and insurance easier to understand. Speaking with someone trained in helping you complete or review these documents is very important if you are not already familiar with them. If the first person you speak to can't explain things in terms you understand, or is impatient with you, please find someone else. There are good professionals out there who truly understand what it means to care for someone with dementia or other serious health issues and are ready to provide compassionate support for you and your loved one.

Essential Legal Documents for Alzheimer's Care

Handling legal documentation may be far from what you imagined when you first stepped into the role of a caregiver. Yet, understanding and organizing these documents is crucial for respecting your loved one's care preferences and wishes throughout the progression of Alzheimer's. Documents such as wills, durable powers of attorney for healthcare and finances, living wills, and advance directives form the backbone of effective legal planning, each serving a distinct purpose.

- **Trusts and Wills** outline how an individual's possessions and assets are distributed according to their wishes after they pass away.
- **Durable Power of Attorney for Finances** (DPOA for Finances) allows a designated person to manage your finances and make decisions about financial matters on your behalf when you are no longer able to do so.
- **Durable Power of Attorney for Healthcare** (DPOA for Healthcare) designates the person who will make medical decisions when you are unable to. Sometimes, backups are

listed as well, in the order they would serve. This may be documented in a Trust, a Living Will, or an Advance Healthcare Directive.

- **Living wills** provide specific instructions regarding your loved one's medical treatment preferences in scenarios where they might not be able to express these wishes verbally.

- **Advance directives** are documents that outline a person's wishes for end-of-life care, including "do-not-resuscitate" (DNR) orders. These directives specify when and under what circumstances they want to receive life-saving measures. Having an advance directive helps guide the family and medical team in creating a care plan that respects their loved one's preferences.

- **POLST Forms** (Physicians Orders for Life Sustaining Treatment) are legal documents that physicians and medical teams are required to follow when providing care. These forms can vary by state, but their primary purpose is to ensure that a person's healthcare decisions are respected no matter where they are. POLST forms often cover critical choices like whether to perform CPR, intubate, provide tube feeding, use long term life sustaining treatments, and when to hospitalize a patient. To see what forms are used in your state, visit https://polst.org/state-polst-programs/.

These documents serve as the voice for your loved one when they are no longer able to speak for themselves, reflecting their values and preferences. Creating these documents isn't just a legal process; it's a deeply personal one that requires careful thought and consideration.

Setting Up Legal Documents

Wills, Trusts, and Durable Power of Attorney for Finances

Setting up legal documents like wills, trusts, and durable power of attorney for finances typically involves several key steps. First, consult with legal professionals who specialize in elder law or estate planning. These experts can provide personalized guidance, assist with complex legal matters, and ensure that all documents are legally valid. To find a reputable attorney, seek recommendations from friends, family, or local Alzheimer's associations.

Living Will, Advance Healthcare Directive, Durable Power of Attorney for Healthcare, POLST

Several documents allow you to specify your medical wishes and designate who will make medical decisions on your behalf if you're unable to. Some of these documents, like POLST forms, are legally binding orders that physicians must follow, while others simply outline your preferences. Working with both legal and medical professionals can help you determine which documents are important for you to complete and clarify the medical implications of each decision. For instance, you can specify a Durable Power of Attorney for Healthcare in a trust, will, living will, or advance healthcare directive.

Preparing these documents involves detailed and sometimes difficult discussions about your loved one's wishes for their care and the management of their affairs. This process may require multiple conversations where you gently guide them through various scenarios and help them decide how they want these situations handled. It requires sensitivity and patience, as it can be emotional to think about these topics.

Is it Too Late for a Will?

You may be concerned that your loved one is no longer competent to make a will. In most states, competency to execute a will requires not much more than knowing what they own and who their heirs are. Consulting with a professional is key to ensure that there is ample evidence of the required competency and that all legal requirements for the will to be valid are satisfied.

If your loved one cannot execute a will, all is not lost. All states have laws in place for such circumstances, intended to be in alignment with how most people would dispose of their property in a properly executed will. Many assets can pass without a will through beneficiary designations and shared ownership. The first step in planning for your loved one's Will is typically to inventory their assets and, with the help of professionals, determine which assets must be addressed in the will and which will bypass it entirely.

Choosing a Durable Power of Attorney

A durable power of attorney authorizes the person to act for the "principal" (your loved one) in all relevant matters. The primary documents that are key here are:

- Durable Power of Attorney for Healthcare (DPOA for Healthcare)
- Durable Power of Attorney for Finances (DPOA for Finances)

Choosing the right person to act as a durable power of attorney places enormous trust in that person. This individual will be responsible for making decisions that affect all aspects of your loved one's life. The ideal candidate is trustworthy and understands your loved one's wishes and values. They should be willing to serve in this capacity and capable of making tough decisions under stressful conditions.

When discussing this role with them, be clear about the responsibilities involved and gauge their comfort and ability to commit to this role long-term. Discuss scenarios they might need to handle, especially end-of-life decisions, and ensure they have all the information needed to make informed decisions that align with your loved one's desires. It's also essential that the person appointed to help with the DPOA is authorized under federal law to access private health information (PHI) about your loved one or can legally assist with any financial matters.

> *Scott's mother was transferred from the hospital to a skilled nursing facility after a fall, and he was told that she would need more caregiving support when she got home as her Alzheimer's was progressing. His four siblings and their mother agreed that because Scott lived just a few hours away and could work a flexible schedule, Scott would assume primary responsibility for her care. Scott was designated as the nursing home's primary contact for questions and concerns, and under HIPAA, Scott was authorized to discuss his mother's care with her doctors and other healthcare providers. In return, Scott kept his siblings up to date on their mother's condition through regular group emails. Scott's mother had a strong advocate for her care, so she could go home sooner, and all her children felt informed and grateful for the responsibility Scott had taken on.*

Understanding Long-Term Care Costs

W hen we talk about the costs of long-term care for people with Alzheimer's, we're looking at several key areas, including in-home care, residential care facilities, medications, and emergency care. In-home care expenses can vary widely, depending on the amount of care required. Part-time help from a home health aide might be significantly less expensive than full-time care.

On average, in the United States, in-home caregivers can range from $15 to $25 per hour in areas with a low cost of living, and $30 to $45 per hour in high-cost areas. Residential care facilities often range from $3,000 to more than $10,000 per month, depending on the level of care, amenities provided, and cost of living in your area. Medication costs also add up, especially as the disease progresses and more medications are needed to manage symptoms and related health issues. Emergency care, which might include hospital stays or emergency medical interventions, can create unexpected financial burdens.

Managing Costs

Managing these costs starts with a solid understanding of the insurance coverages available. Medicare and Medicaid can often be confusing for many caregivers. Original Medicare, the federal health insurance program for seniors, typically covers doctor visits, preventive services, and hospital stays, and short-term home health care but does not cover long-term care in a residential facility. Medicare Advantage and Medicare Supplemental Plans (Medigap) are additional plans to provide insurance for medications, routine exams, and other services that Medicare does not cover. Check out https://medicare.gov for more information.

Medicaid is health care coverage administered by states for qualifying individuals. It may cover long-term care for individuals with income and assets below certain thresholds and who meet certain medical criteria. Check out https://medicaid.gov for more information about the program and links for your state specific information.

Understanding these programs requires a thorough knowledge of eligibility requirements and benefits coverage. It's often helpful to consult with a financial advisor and social worker who specialize in elder care to manage the complexities of these programs.

Long-Term Care Insurance

Long-term care insurance is another integral component of financial planning for Alzheimer's care. This type of insurance is designed to cover services that Medicare and other health insurance programs typically do not, such as extended nursing home stays and non-medical home care.

When choosing a long-term care insurance policy, consider factors such as coverage limits, what triggers coverage, inflation protection, and the reputation of the insurance provider. Policies can vary significantly, and the right choice depends on your loved one's needs and your financial circumstances. It's a good idea to purchase a policy sooner rather than later, as premiums increase with age and coverage is cheaper when purchased at a younger age.

Financial Assistance Programs

Looking into different financial assistance programs is incredibly valuable. Various federal, state, and local programs can help alleviate some of the financial burdens of Alzheimer's care. These might include veteran's benefits, state-specific Medicaid programs, or community-based programs offering subsidies for respite care or home modifications, and grant programs for other care needs. Information on these programs is usually available through local Alzheimer's associations, Area Agencies on Aging, or through an eldercare planner. Also explore organizations dedicated to providing support for certain communities that have experienced significant past trauma, such as Holocaust Survivors.

Budgeting for Alzheimer's Care

Budgeting for Alzheimer's care involves strategic planning and sometimes tough decision-making. Start by creating a detailed budget that outlines all potential costs, from daily care needs to future expenses. Regularly review and adjust this budget as care needs evolve and financial situations change.

If managing these financial responsibilities becomes overwhelming, consider working with a financial planner who has experience in elder care. They can offer invaluable guidance on protecting assets, planning for future expenses, and maintaining your loved one's financial security throughout the progression of Alzheimer's.

Understanding the costs involved in long-term care and how to handle insurance options, financial assistance programs, and budgeting can create a more stable and sustainable care environment for your loved one. Every step you take in managing these financial aspects ensures your loved one receives the quality care they deserve without compromising their financial well-being, or yours.

Section Six
Innovations in Alzheimer's Care

Nancy's family was known to have a rare genetic disease called cardiac amyloidosis, which creates an overproduction of the amyloid protein. Her family usually discovered the disease when heart problems showed up, but with hindsight, the Alzheimer's symptoms often showed up first. Nancy's uncle had died from heart related complications of the disease, because at the time, there was no medication or therapy to slow the production of the amyloid protein. When Nancy's sister, Destiny, became ill, a new medication was available that slowed the amyloid protein production. It improved her heart functioning and appeared to reduce the severity of some of her Alzheimer's symptoms, like anxiety and agitation.
Please note: It did not reverse Destiny's Alzheimer's symptoms, but gave the family some breathing room for a short time.

This book has already incorporated practical research findings throughout the caregiver strategies listed in the Sections Two and

Three. These are the strategies that relate to findings around diet, cognitive exercises, physical activity and social engagement, amongst others. As research continues, it is helpful to stay current on new trends to help manage the symptoms and slow the cognitive decline.

.

Alzheimer's Research

R esearch on Alzheimer's is promising, yet always changing, and constantly pushing the boundaries of our understanding of this complex disease. Recent breakthroughs in drug development offer new hope to individuals and families dealing with Alzheimer's. These innovations focus on addressing biological processes behind the disease, such as amyloid plaques and tau proteins, which are key contributors to the cognitive decline seen in people with Alzheimer's.

The concept of neuroplasticity, or the brain's ability to reorganize itself by forming new neural connections, is gaining increased attention. This adaptability forms the basis for cognitive rehabilitation and brain training programs, which aim to improve or maintain cognitive function in people with Alzheimer's. Programs that stimulate mental activity, challenge the brain, and encourage new skills have shown potential in slowing cognitive decline. These therapies, often used alongside traditional treatments, can be tailored to the specific needs and capabilities of each person, making them versatile tools in managing Alzheimer's.

Early and accurate diagnoses are vital for effective management of Alzheimer's. Innovations in this area include blood tests that can detect biomarkers associated with the disease, such as specific proteins indicating the presence of amyloid plaques in the brain. These tests are becoming more sophisticated and accessible, providing a less invasive and more cost-effective method for diagnosis than traditional brain imaging techniques. Further, advancements in imaging technologies, such as PET scans, allow researchers and doctors to observe the brain in greater detail, improving their ability to diagnose Alzheimer's earlier and more accurately.

Research into lifestyle factors that influence the risk of developing Alzheimer's is also yielding valuable insights. Studies on diet, exercise, cognitive training, and social engagement suggest that daily habits significantly affect our risk for developing the disease. Diets rich in fruits, vegetables, whole grains, and healthy fats, such as the Mediterranean diet, have been linked to a lower risk of cognitive decline. Regular physical activity, mental stimulation through new skills or hobbies, and maintaining strong social connections all contribute to brain health. This body of research supports the idea that while genetics and biology play significant roles, there are actions we can take to potentially reduce our risk of Alzheimer's.

The more we continue to learn about these exciting research areas, the more our approach to caring for and preventing Alzheimer's improves. Each new discovery helps us understand this complex disease better and boosts our ability to offer more effective, personalized, and compassionate care. The future of Alzheimer's research is looking bright, thanks to ongoing innovation and a relentless search for knowledge.

Staying Updated on Research and News

In the fast-evolving field of Alzheimer's research, staying informed isn't just about keeping up with the latest news—it's about empowering yourself with knowledge that can change your approach to caregiving. Imagine having insights that could predict changes, manage symptoms more effectively, or even slow down the progression of the disease. That's the power of keeping up with the latest advancements in Alzheimer's research.

Sources for Current Research

It's imperative to know where to find reliable and up-to-date information on Alzheimer's research. Start with respected medical journals like the *Journal of Alzheimer's Disease* or *Alzheimer's & Dementia*, which publish peer-reviewed articles and breakthrough studies. Websites of reputable Alzheimer's organizations such as the Alzheimer's Association and Alzheimer's Foundation of America are also treasure troves of updated research, news, and resources. The UK Dementia Research Institute is involved in cutting edge research on Dementia. Health news websites like WebMD or Medscape also provide easy-to-understand summaries of the latest research findings. Make sure to choose sources that are well-respected and frequently updated to reflect the latest scientific discoveries.

Understanding Research Findings

Medical research can seem overwhelming with its complex language and statistics. However, understanding these can significantly impact how you apply this knowledge to everyday caregiving. Focus on terms commonly used in Alzheimer's research like 'neuroplasticity,' 'cognitive decline,' and 'biomarkers.' Knowing what these terms mean can help you grasp the broader implications of the studies. Pay attention to how studies are structured and their sample sizes, as these factors can affect the reliability of the findings. Smaller studies or those without control groups might not provide strong evidence, so consider these aspects when interpreting results.

Integrating New Knowledge into Care

Every piece of research has the potential to change care practices. For example, if recent studies suggest that certain diets or exercises can slow cognitive decline, try incorporating these into your daily routine. If a study highlights the benefits of a Mediterranean diet for improving cognitive function, consider gradually introducing more fruits, vegetables, nuts, and whole grains into your loved one's diet. It's about taking new insights and making them part of your caregiving approach to improve your loved one's quality of life.

Networking with Professionals

Building connections with healthcare professionals and researchers can provide invaluable insights and advice for navigating Alzheimer's care. Attend conferences, seminars, and workshops dedicated to Alzheimer's research and care. Many of these events now offer virtual attendance options, making them more accessible. Engaging in these settings allows you to ask questions directly to experts, stay ahead of treatment trends, and bring back helpful strategies that can be adapted to your caregiving situation. Moreover, these networks can form a supportive community from which you can draw strength and knowledge, reminding you that you're not alone in this challenge.

Stepping into the Role of an Informed Caregiver

Being an informed caregiver can truly redefine the care journey for both you and your loved one. By staying updated, understanding the research, applying new knowledge, and networking with professionals, you equip yourself with the tools to approach Alzheimer's with a proactive and informed approach. This ongoing learning process not only enriches your caregiving practices but also brings hope and empowerment to a journey that can often feel uncertain.

Staying updated on Alzheimer's research and applying innovative caregiving techniques and technologies, allows us to proactively implement the best that science and wisdom have to offer.

Section Seven

Honoring Your Loved One's Legacy

Lisa knew that her mother loved the ocean, the museums, and the gardens she had frequented as a child. As her mother aged, she found it difficult to go to these places on her own, so she simply stopped. Lisa realized she wanted to create some special memories with her mother before her mother was no longer around. So, together with her three sons, Lisa planned trips with her mother, taking her to all of her favorite places. They took pictures and videos on every trip, savoring each moment of their time together. When Lisa's mother died, she used some of the pictures and videos for the memorial service. As Lisa watched the videos, she realized she hadn't just captured memories of her mother but had preserved family moments that her children and future generations would have as well.

Caring for a loved one with Alzheimer's is a journey filled with countless challenges, tender moments, and precious memories. As a caregiver, you carry the weight of making each day meaningful, all while grappling with the reality that time is limited. This chapter is here to remind you that, amid the daily tasks and emotional ups and downs, there's still room for beauty, connection, and legacy. Creating memories are not just about the past—they're a way to enrich the present and honor your loved one's life story, even as their memories fade.

Preserving Memories

The ideas shared in this chapter aren't complicated or time-consuming—they're about small, intentional actions that can be woven into your everyday life. From crafting memory books to recording favorite stories, these suggestions are designed to help you create keepsakes that will hold your loved one's spirit long after they're gone.

So, take a moment. Slow down. The time you spend today capturing these memories will be the threads that tie the past to the future, for you, your loved ones, and generations to come. By making these moments a priority now, you're not just preserving the past—you're creating a legacy of love that will endure, no matter what the future holds.

Creating Memory Books and Boxes

One of the most heartfelt projects you can undertake is creating memory books or boxes. These collections of photos, mementos, and notes serve as a tangible link to the past, not only for your loved one but for the entire family. Start by selecting a variety of photos that capture different stages of their life—childhood, young adulthood, major life events, recent years—and include keepsakes that hold special significance, such as a pressed flower from a family vacation or a ticket stub from a favorite concert.

Assembling these items can be a comforting activity for your loved one, offering them a sense of connection to familiar times. Looking through old photos and discussing the stories behind these mementos can stimulate their memory and provide enjoyable moments of recall. For family members, especially younger ones who might not remember earlier times, these books and boxes provide an opportunity for connection and learning, sparking conversations and providing deeper insights into the family history.

The therapeutic benefits of this activity are profound. For your loved one, it reinforces identity and continuity in their life story, which can be grounding in moments of confusion. For caregivers and family members, it's a way to engage with your loved one beyond the disease, remembering and celebrating their full life and contributions.

Recording Oral Histories

Another powerful way to preserve your loved one's legacy is by recording oral histories. This can be especially meaningful if your loved one is still able to communicate verbally. Set up a comfortable, quiet space to make these recordings, ensuring minimal background noise. Use a simple audio recorder or smartphone app and prepare a list of prompts to help guide the conversation if needed. These might include questions about their favorite childhood memories, significant life milestones, or advice they'd like to pass on to future generations.

Approach these sessions with flexibility and patience. There may be days when your loved one feels more communicative than others, and that's okay. The goal is to capture the essence of their experiences and thoughts in their own words, providing a priceless artifact for the family. These recordings can be especially cherished, offering a way to hear their voice and revisit their stories even after they're no longer able to tell them.

Consider Legacy Projects

Legacy projects, such as planting a garden, compiling a family recipe book, or crafting a quilt, provide a sense of purpose and continuity for individuals with Alzheimer's. These projects can be therapeutic, offering a focus for activity and a way to contribute something lasting to the family or community. For instance, planting a garden can be a multi-sensory activity that ties memories to the physical world. As the seasons change, it becomes a living symbol of growth and renewal, reflective of your loved one's life.

When choosing a project, think about what aligns best with your loved one's interests and abilities. Compiling a family recipe book might be perfect for someone who loves cooking, providing a chance to pass down cherished recipes and associated stories. Each page can be a celebration of family gatherings and shared meals, enriched with personal notes and photos.

Using Technology to Share and Preserve Memories

In today's age, technology offers incredible tools for sharing and preserving memories. Online photo albums can be easily created and shared with family members across the globe, ensuring everyone has access to the cherished moments captured over the years. Blogs and other storytelling platforms allow for a more narrative approach, where photos and stories can be combined to create a meaningful record of your loved one's life.

When using these tools, pay careful attention to privacy settings to make sure your family's memories are shared only with those you choose. Many platforms allow you to set passwords or create private groups, offering a secure space for family members to contribute memories and comments. This can be particularly comforting for family members who may not be able to visit often, providing them a way to stay connected and participate in preserving the family legacy.

In each of these endeavors, from creating memory books to recording oral histories, the focus is not just on preservation but on celebration. It's about putting together something enduring and meaningful, a reminder of the life and love shared with your loved one. As you embark on these projects, remember that each step taken, each memory preserved, strengthens the bonds of family and honors your loved one's profound journey through Alzheimer's.

Keeping the Journey Alive

Now that you have the tools to care for your loved one with confidence and compassion, it's time to share what you've learned and help others find the same support.

By leaving your honest review on Amazon, you'll guide other caregivers toward the help they need. Your voice matters—it can be the light that leads another reader to the information and encouragement they're searching for.

Thank you for your support. The heart of caregiving stays strong when we pass on what we know. You're helping keep this journey alive for all of us.

Scan the QR code below and leave your review:

Closing Thoughts

As our journey through the pages of this handbook comes to an end, I want to take a moment to reflect on the path we've traveled together. From the uncertain first steps when Alzheimer's first touched our lives to becoming more empowered and resourceful caregivers, we've navigated challenges and found moments of deep connection.

Remember, caring for a loved one with Alzheimer's is a true act of empathy and compassion. It asks us to step into the shoes of another person, to see the world as they do, and to respond with patience and understanding. This journey changes us, teaching us the true meaning of resilience and the power of a gentle touch or kind word.

The Secret to Alzheimer's Dementia Care lies in the three-fold integration of knowledge, adaptability, and self-care.

First, knowledge gives you confidence in your caregiving abilities. You learn what to expect—even if it means never fully knowing what to expect—and how to handle constant changes. You understand that trial and error are part of the process, and just when you think you've finally figured it out, there will be something new to learn. By replacing fear of the unknown with curiosity, you develop emotional strength, allowing you to offer compassionate care and appreciate the meaningful moments at each stage.

Second, adaptability means meeting your loved one where they are, not where you want them to be. It's about staying attuned to the subtle shifts in their behavior and cognition and being flexible enough to adjust your routines and approach as their needs evolve.

Finally, the glue that holds everything together is prioritizing your own well-being through self-care. We've discussed various strategies to manage stress, seek support, and take care of yourself because the quality of your caregiving ultimately depends on how well you care for yourself.

I encourage you to build a strong support network. Connect with healthcare professionals, join support groups, and share your experiences and strategies. There's great strength in community, and by connecting with others, you not only gain more resources but also contribute to the collective knowledge of Alzheimer's care.

In the midst of all this, I acknowledge the emotional complexities you face—the grief, the loss, and the evolving dynamics of your relationship with your loved one. These feelings are a natural part of your caregiving journey; you're not alone in feeling them.

Despite the challenges, there are always moments of joy to be found. Celebrate small victories, cherish quiet moments of connection, and hold onto the memories you create each day. These moments are precious lights in the journey of caregiving.

So, there you have it, The Secret to Alzheimer's Dementia Care.

Consider advocating for increased Alzheimer's research and improved support services. Together, our voices can create significant change, improving Alzheimer's care for those who follow in our footsteps. Your journey is unique, but together, we walk a common path.

As we part ways in this book, remember, you are not alone. Your dedication, love, and resilience are seen and deeply appreciated. May you continue to find strength, hope, and courage as you move forward. Think of this not just as an ending, but as an invitation to reach out, share your story, and keep learning and growing. Keep the conversation going—your experiences and insights are invaluable in building a more understanding and supportive community for every Alzheimer's caregiver.

Thank you for your trust, your time, and your commitment to caring for those who once cared for us, or impacted our lives, in a special way. Here's to more good days, meaningful moments, and continued support along the way.

Peace and Blessings,

Renée

References

A Place for Mom. (2023). 9 free apps for caregivers. *A Place for Mom.* https://www. aplaceformom.com/caregiver-resources/articles/family-caregiver-apps

Achterberg, W. P., Pieper, M. J., van Dalen-Kok, A. H., de Waal, M. W., Husebo, B. S., Lautenbacher, S., & Scherder, E. J. (2013). Pain management in patients with dementia. *Clinical Interventions in Aging, 8,* 1471–1482. https://www.ncbi.nlm. nih.gov/pmc/articles/PMC3817007/

AgeTech Collaborative. (2023). Smart home technology for older adults. *AgeTech Collaborative.* https://agetechcollaborative.org/custom_resource/smart-home-tech-for-older-adults/

AgingCare. (n.d.). Expert advice: How to choose a mobility aid for a senior. *Aging-Care.* https://www.agingcare.com/articles/expert-advice-how-to-choose-a-mobil ity-aid-190138.htm

AIXR. (2021). How virtual reality can transform dementia care. *AIXR.* https://aixr. org/insights/how-virtual-reality-can-transform-dementia-care/

Al-Shaqi, R. A., Mourshed, M., & Rezgui, Y. (2023). The use of visual methods to support communication with people living with dementia. *Sensors, 23*(4), 1245. https://www.ncbi.nlm.nih.gov/pmc/articles/PMC10033830/

Almutary, H., Alomari, H., Alonazi, A., Bani-Issa, W., Othman, N., & Aldebasi, T. M. (2021). Approach to management of wandering in dementia. *International Journal of Environmental Research and Public Health, 18*(21), 11459. https:// www.ncbi.nlm.nih.gov/pmc/articles/PMC8543604/

Alzheimer's Association. (n.d.). Alzheimer's & dementia training & education center. *Alzheimer's Association.* https://training.alz.org/

Alzheimer's Association. (n.d.). Approaching Alzheimer's: First responder training. *Alzheimer's Association.* https://www.alz.org/professionals/first-responders

Alzheimer's Association. (n.d.). Caregiver stress. *Alzheimer's Association.* https:// www.alz.org/help-support/caregiving/caregiver-health/caregiver-stress

Alzheimer's Association. (n.d.). Communication. *Alzheimer's Association.* https:// www.alz.org/help-support/caregiving/daily-care/communications

Alzheimer's Association. (n.d.). Dementia care practice recommendations. *Alzheimer's Association.* https://www.alz.org/professionals/professional-providers/dementia_care_practice_recommendations

Alzheimer's Association. (n.d.). Financial and legal planning for caregivers. *Alzheimer's Association.* https://www.alz.org/help-support/caregiving/financial-legal-planning

Alzheimer's Association. (n.d.). Food & eating. *Alzheimer's Association*. https://www.alz.org/help-support/caregiving/daily-care/food-eating

Alzheimer's Association. (n.d.). Grief and loss as Alzheimer's progresses. *Alzheimer's Association*. https://www.alz.org/help-support/caregiving/caregiver-health/grief-loss-as-alzheimers-progresses

Alzheimer's Association. (n.d.). Home safety. *Alzheimer's Association*. https://www.alz.org/help-support/caregiving/safety/home-safety

Alzheimer's Association. (n.d.). Models of care case studies. *Alzheimer's Association*. https://www.alz.org/professionals/health-systems-medical-professionals/management/case-studies

Alzheimer's Association. (n.d.). Support groups. *Alzheimer's Association*. https://www.alz.org/help-support/community/support-groups

Alzheimer's Disease International. (n.d.). Organising events for awareness raising and fundraising. *Alzheimer's Disease International*. https://www.alzint.org/resource/organising-events-for-awareness-raising-and-fundraising/

Alzheimer's Foundation of America. (n.d.). Alzheimer's and dementia support groups. *Alzheimer's Foundation of America*. https://alzfdn.org/caregiving-resources/alzheimers-and-dementia-support-groups/

Alzheimer's Impact Movement. (2019). Medicaid eligibility and people with Alzheimer's. *Alzheimer's Association*. https://portal.alzimpact.org/media/serve/id/5d23aed5e8dfa

Alzheimer's Impact Movement. (2023). Progress in the fight against Alzheimer's. *Alzheimer's Association*. https://alzimpact.org/our-successes

Alzheimer's Society. (n.d.). How technology can help. *Alzheimer's Society*. https://www.alzheimers.org.uk/get-support/staying-independent/how-technology-can-help

Alzheimer's Society. (n.d.). How to support children and young people when a person has dementia. *Alzheimer's Society*. https://www.alzheimers.org.uk/get-support/daily-living/supporting-children-young-people-dementia

Alzheimer's Society. (n.d.). Non-verbal communication and dementia. *Alzheimer's Society*. https://www.alzheimers.org.uk/about-dementia/symptoms-and-diagnosis/symptoms/non-verbal-communication-and-dementia

Being in the Moment. (n.d.). About us. https://beinginthemoment.org/about-us/

Bethesda Health. (2021). Long-distance caregiving made easier with technology. *Bethesda Health*. https://bethesdahealth.org/blog/2021/11/02/long-distance-caregiving-made-easier-technology/

Black, K., & Reynolds, S. L. (2013). Facilitating end-of-life decision-making strategies for people with dementia: The role of proxy decision-makers. *The Gerontologist, 53*(2), 236-245. https://www.ncbi.nlm.nih.gov/pmc/articles/PMC3732104/

Brodaty, H., & Donkin, M. (2011). Effect of educational and supportive strategies on the well-being of family caregivers of people with dementia. *Journal of the Amer-

ican Geriatrics Society, 59(7), 1200-1207. https://pubmed.ncbi.nlm.nih.gov/22026322/

Callaghan, P. (2004). Exercise for mental health. *Primary Care Companion to The Journal of Clinical Psychiatry, 6*(3), 104-111. https://www.ncbi.nlm.nih.gov/pmc/articles/PMC1470658/

Care Partners. (2023). Memory care vs. in-home care for dementia: What's the difference? *Care Part*ners. https://carepartners.us/memory-care-vs-in-home-care-for-dementia-whats-the-difference/

Care.com. (n.d.). Caregiver guilt is normal: Expert tips for coping. *Care.com*. https://www.care.com/c/tips-for-managing-caregiver-guilt/

CareBand. (n.d.). CareBand – Location-based health and safety solutions. *CareBand*. https://carebandremembers.com

Caregiving.com. (n.d.). Easing movement 101: A caregiver's guide to support and mobility assistance. *Caregiving.com*. https://www.caregiving.com/content/easing-movement-101-a-caregivers-guide-to-support-and-mobility-assistance

Chamine, S. (2012). *Positive intelligence: Why only 20% of teams and individuals achieve their true potential and how you can achieve yours.* Greenleaf Book Group Press.

DailyCaring. (n.d.). 10 expert time management tips for caregivers. *DailyCaring*. https://dailycaring.com/10-best-time-management-tips-for-caregivers-from-a-true-expert/

Firth, J., Stubbs, B., Vancampfort, D., Schuch, F., Rosenbaum, S., Ward, P. B., & Curtis, J. (2018). Physical exercise enhances neuroplasticity and delays Alzheimer's disease progression: A systematic review of randomized controlled trials. *BMC Geriatrics, 18*(1), 193. https://www.ncbi.nlm.nih.gov/pmc/articles/PMC6296269/

Freedom Care. (n.d.). The 40 best caregiver training programs. *Freedom Care*. https://freedomcare.com/caregiver-training/

Harvard Health Publishing. (2022). Foods that fight inflammation. *Harvard Medical School*. https://www.health.harvard.edu/staying-healthy/foods-that-fight-inflammation

Healthline. (2022). Memory care: Services, benefits, and cost. *Healthline*. https://www.healthline.com/health/what-is-memory-care

Iwelunmor, J., Newsome, V., & Airhihenbuwa, C. O. (2018). Cultural competency in dementia care: An African American perspective. *Journal of Cross-Cultural Gerontology, 33*(3), 321-340. https://www.ncbi.nlm.nih.gov/pmc/articles/PMC5935110/

Kuller, L. H., & Lopez, O. L. (2019). Alzheimer's disease – Why we need early diagnosis. *Frontiers in Aging Neuroscience, 11*, 263. https://www.ncbi.nlm.nih.gov/pmc/articles/PMC6935598/

Ledford, H. (2023). How CRISPR gene editing could help treat Alzheimer's. *Nature*. https://www.nature.com/articles/d41586-023-03931-5

Long Island Alzheimer's and Dementia Center. (n.d.). Adaptive devices for persons with dementia. *Long Island Alzheimer's and Dementia Center.* https://www.lide mentia.org/adaptive-devices-dementia/

Mayo Clinic. (2023). Alzheimer's stages: How the disease progresses. *Mayo Clinic.* https://www.mayoclinic.org/diseases-conditions/alzheimers-disease/in-depth/ alzheimers-stages/art-20048448

Mayo Clinic. (2023). Mindfulness exercises. *Mayo Clinic.* https://www.mayoclinic.org/ healthy-lifestyle/consumer-health/in-depth/mindfulness-exercises/art-20046356

Mayo Foundation for Medical Education and Research. (2023, June 7). Alzheimer's stages: How the disease progresses. *Mayo Clinic.* https://www.mayoclinic.org/ diseases-conditions/alzheimers-disease/in-depth/alzheimers-stages/art-20048448

Medical News Today. (2023). Dementia and power of attorney: What to know. *Medical News Today.* https://www.medicalnewstoday.com/articles/how-to-change-power-of-attorney-for-someone-with-dementia

Muscular Dystrophy Association. (n.d.). Meals for easy swallowing. *Muscular Dystrophy Association.* https://www.mda.org/sites/default/files/publications/ Meals_Easy_Swallowing_P-508.pdf

National Council on Aging. (2024). The 7 best medical alert systems with GPS in 2024. *National Council on Aging.* https://www.ncoa.org/adviser/medical-alert-systems/best-medical-alert-systems-with-gps/

National Council on Aging. (n.d.). Long-term care insurance and memory care. *National Council on Aging.* https://www.ncoa.org/article/does-long-term-care-insurance-cover-memory-care-a-comprehensive-guide

National Institute on Aging. (2021). Legal and financial planning for people living with dementia [Fact sheet]. *National Institutes of Health.* https://order.nia.nih. gov/sites/default/files/2021-01/legal-financial-planning-dementia-factsheet.pdf

National Institute on Aging. (2022). Alzheimer's caregiving: Changes in communication skills. *National Institutes of Health.* https://www.nia.nih.gov/health/ alzheimers-changes-behavior-and-communication/alzheimers-caregiving-changes-communication

National Institute on Aging. (2022). Managing personality and behavior changes in Alzheimer's. *National Institutes of Health.* https://www.nia.nih.gov/health/ alzheimers-changes-behavior-and-communication/managing-personality-and-behavior-changes

National Institute on Aging. (2022). What do we know about diet and prevention of Alzheimer's disease? *National Institutes of Health.* https://www.nia.nih.gov/ health/alzheimers-and-dementia/what-do-we-know-about-diet-and-prevention-alzheimers-disease

National Institute on Aging. (2023). Alzheimer's disease: Common medical problems. *National Institutes of Health.* https://www.nia.nih.gov/health/alzheimers-caregiv ing/alzheimers-disease-common-medical-problems

National Institute on Aging. (2023). Coping with agitation and aggression in Alzheimer's disease. *National Institutes of Health*. https://www.nia.nih.gov/ health/alzheimers-changes-behavior-and-communication/coping-agitation-and-aggression-alzheimers

National Institute on Aging. (2023). Helping family and friends understand Alzheimer's disease. *National Institutes of Health*. https://www.nia.nih.gov/ health/alzheimers-and-relationships/helping-family-and-friends-understand-alzheimers-disease

National Institute on Aging. (2023). Staying physically active with Alzheimer's. *National Institutes of Health*. https://www.nia.nih.gov/health/exercise-and-physi cal-activity/staying-physically-active-alzheimers

National Institute on Aging. (2023). Wandering and Alzheimer's disease. *National Institutes of Health*. https://www.nia.nih.gov/health/alzheimers-changes-behav ior-and-communication/wandering-and-alzheimers-disease

NHS. (2023). How to make your home dementia friendly. *NHS*. https://www.nhs. uk/conditions/dementia/living-with-dementia/home-environment/

Osman, S. E., Tischler, V., & Schneider, J. (2016). The arts as a medium for care and self-care in dementia: Arguments and evidence. *International Journal of Environmental Research and Public Health, 13*(9), 926. https://www.ncbi.nlm.nih.gov/ pmc/articles/PMC6025004/

Salmon Health. (2021). Sensory stimulation for older adults with dementia. *Salmon Health*. https://salmonhealth.com/sensory-stimulation-for-older-adults-with-dementia/

SilverSneakers. (2022). The best online support groups for Alzheimer's caregivers. *SilverSneakers*. https://www.silversneakers.com/blog/the-best-online-support-groups-for-alzheimers-caregivers/

Span, M., Hettinga, M., Vernooij-Dassen, M., Eefsting, J., & Smits, C. (2016). Evaluation of the digital Alzheimer center: Testing usability and usefulness of an online portal for patients with dementia and their caregivers. *JMIR Research Protocols, 5*(3), e144. https://www.ncbi.nlm.nih.gov/pmc/articles/PMC4974452/

Teepa Snow. (2023). Dementia care: 6 tips to overcome challenging family dynamics. *Teepa Snow*. https://teepasnow.com/blog/dementia-care-6-tips-to-overcome-chal lenging-family-dynamics/

van der Wardt, V., Hancox, J., Gonczi, T., Pulford, R., & Mitchell, D. (2020). Potential benefits of physical activity in mild cognitive impairment and dementia. *Progress in Neurology and Psychiatry, 24*(1), 23-28. https://www.ncbi.nlm.nih. gov/pmc/articles/PMC7037481/

WebMD. (n.d.). Brain exercises for dementia: How they help the mind. *WebMD*. https://www.webmd.com/alzheimers/preventing-dementia-brain-exercises

WebMD. (n.d.). Foods that help tame stress. *WebMD*. https://www.webmd.com/ diet/ss/slideshow-diet-for-stress-management

Wirecutter. (2023). The best medical alert systems. *The New York Times*. https://www.nytimes.com/wirecutter/reviews/the-best-medical-alert-systems/

Yale Medicine. (2023). Lecanemab, the new Alzheimer's treatment. *Yale Medicine*. https://www.yalemedicine.org/news/lecanemab-leqembi-new-alzheimers-drug

Zhang, Y., Cai, J., An, L., Hui, F., Ren, T., Ma, H., & Zhao, Q. (2017). Music therapy in the treatment of dementia: A systematic review and meta-analysis. *Frontiers in Psychology, 8*, 748. https://www.ncbi.nlm.nih.gov/pmc/articles/PMC7248378/

Zhang, Y., Sun, Y., Zhang, S., Li, W., & Zhang, L. (2023). Water intake, hydration status, and 2-year changes in cognitive performance in older adults. *Nutrients, 15*(2), 351. https://www.ncbi.nlm.nih.gov/pmc/articles/PMC9993798/

www.ingramcontent.com/pod-product-compliance
Lightning Source LLC
Chambersburg PA
CBHW032056020426
42335CB00011B/365